Anchored in hope:

A journey of healing from chronic fatigue syndrome

Dana Harlow

First published 2023. Revised 2024.

DISCLAIMER
This book is not intended for giving medical advice. This book is the personal experience of the author. The author takes no responsibility for adverse consequences of a reader applying what they have read.

Bible quotes:

Other sources:
Bridgeman, Philip. (2004). *Daniel's Diet.* PK Self Publishers.
Bridgeman, Philip. (2005). *Daniel's Diet Lifestyle.* PK Self Publishers.

Contact the author:
anchored-in-hope@outlook.com

Dedicated to the heroes of this story:

Jesus, the anchor of hope
Mum and Dad who constantly cared
My sister, Rachel, with wisdom beyond her years to feed me the Word
My amazing school friend, Linda, who kept me connected
My Aunty Jody who followed the whispers of the Holy Spirit
And to all those who are navigating an 'incurable' condition
– please hold on to the anchor of hope!

Special thank you to:

Shontelle Hughes for painting and designing the front cover
Julie Townsend for editing
Simon Harlow for editing
Philip Bridgeman for permission to use quotes from his books
Readers for taking the time to read my story
Jesus for being with me every step of the way, for healing me, for compelling me to write this story out

Table of Contents

Introduction

Chronic fatigue is a terrible condition for anyone to have. There seems to be an increasing number of people who are suffering with it. With each of these individuals – maybe you are one of them – I am sure there is a unique story and journey of how chronic fatigue has impacted their lives. It can be a lonely journey and one which is often misunderstood.

This book tells my story, my journey, my experiences with chronic fatigue. I have felt compelled to write this book in order to give people hope and encouragement. Hope that there is a way out. Encouragement that they are not alone. I have sincerely tried to be accurate in everything I have written. I had a significant number of resources to draw on (journals, diaries, calendars, emails, books, university transcript, photos and so on). That being said, conversations and specific moments are hard to remember exactly so they are as accurate as I can recall.

It is my prayer that as you read this book you will grow in faith, be renewed in your mind and be drawn closer to the One who has all the answers – Jesus, the true anchor of hope. (See Hebrews 6:19-20).

Chapter 1:
A day in the life

It was a pleasant summer's afternoon as I sat in the school's Music computer lab finishing off the horn chart for "Beautiful One". Our annual school Presentation Night was just a few days away and this was to be one of the songs. The school year was almost through. I loved that time of year. The warm weather, the fun end of school year activities, the six-week summer holidays just on the horizon. Ahhh. So good.

2006 had been a busy, but good year. At school we had performed a unique production called "A night on Broadway" with a conglomeration of songs from different musicals woven into an original storyline created by one of our English/Drama teachers. I had also been part of a fun trip to Tasmania with the school Stage Band and Concert Band and the crazy four terms crammed into three that is Year 11 was done and dusted. It was definitely hard to fit a year's worth of content and assessment into three terms, but we made it. Now we were nearing the end of the first term of Year 12 which is during the typical Term 4. This was tough because everyone likes to wind down at the end of the year, but in Year 12, it is like Term 1. We needed to get stuck into the Year 12 content and complete our first assessment task for each subject. I had just one assessment left … Extension 1 Maths. I'm not sure why they scheduled it so late in the term, but I suppose it was because we had to have enough time to learn everything before the test.

After getting through the Extension 1 Maths HSC Assessment Task 1 it was definitely feeling like the end of the year. After a few more Presentation Night rehearsals, it was time for the real thing. Presentation Night was a great night of celebration where the whole school (K-12) came together to showcase musical sections, drama performances and present Academic, Sporting and Special Awards to students. It was a big deal. The venue was Wollongong Entertainment Centre and we usually spent all day setting up and rehearsing down there (about an hour's drive from school), and then friends and family would join us for the extravaganza at night. It was so much fun! And Presentation Night 2006 didn't disappoint.   I was asked to play keyboard in the backing band for the massed choir items plus I had fun performing in the Concert Band and Stage Band on the trumpet.

We made the drive back to Sydney and the holidays were just a few days away. I would soon be enjoying Christmas with the family, having relaxing days watching the Test Match cricket and relishing the fun times on the water during our annual Nowra water-skiing holiday with family and friends.

"its (st) in pindyland says:
        Three advantages of AC generators. GO
    Houseparty 06- FROM THE INSIDE OUT!!!!!!! And
the cry of my heart is to bring You praise! says:
        Can be used in conjunction with transformers!
    don't require split-ring commutator = less wear

and tear, can be used for more appliances (and can be rectified to DC anyway)!!!

its (st) in pindyland says:

Think of a better third one

its (st) in pindyland says:

I'm not accepting that one

Houseparty 06- FROM THE INSIDE OUT!!!!!!! And the cry of my heart is to bring You praise! says:

why not?

its (st) in pindyland says:

because there's a better answer out there and i want you to get it

Houseparty 06- FROM THE INSIDE OUT!!!!!!! And the cry of my heart is to bring You praise! says:

fair enough

Houseparty 06- FROM THE INSIDE OUT!!!!!!! And the cry of my heart is to bring You praise! says:

can use 3 phase AC to get a smoother output

its (st) in pindyland says:

good! did you look that up...?

Houseparty 06- FROM THE INSIDE OUT!!!!!!! And the cry of my heart is to bring You praise! says:

i thought of it first then checked it

its (st) in pindyland says:

oh sure sure

Houseparty 06- FROM THE INSIDE OUT!!!!!!! And the cry of my heart is to bring You praise! says:

it's true

its (st) in pindyland says:

what's faraday's law of electromagnetic induction?

Houseparty 06- FROM THE INSIDE OUT!!!!!!! And the cry of my heart is to bring You praise! says:

hey it's my turn to ask u a question!

Houseparty 06- FROM THE INSIDE OUT!!!!!!!! And the cry of my heart is to bring You praise! says:

What are 4 types of scans used for ultrasound?

its (st) in pindyland says:

answer mine first

its (st) in pindyland says:

A scans, B Scans, Sector Scans and phase scans. Come on, that was easy

its (st) in pindyland says:

i havent even studied med physics yet!

Houseparty 06- FROM THE INSIDE OUT!!!!!!!! And the cry of my heart is to bring You praise! says:

ok... i was being nice coz u said ud only studied motors and generators

its (st) in pindyland says:

that's true. but then again that was my focus question to do lol

its (st) in pindyland says:

now answer mine missy

Houseparty 06- FROM THE INSIDE OUT!!!!!!!! And the cry of my heart is to bring You praise! says:

So Faraday's Law- something about cutting lines of flux induces a current in a coil- can remember experiment! clue?

its (st) in pindyland says:

its a formula

its (st) in pindyland says:

you dont get clues in exams lol

Houseparty 06- FROM THE INSIDE OUT!!!!!!!! And the cry of my heart is to bring You praise! says:

E = change in flux over change in time?
its (st) in pindyland says:
emf but yeah
Houseparty 06- FROM THE INSIDE OUT!!!!!!! And the cry of my heart is to bring You praise! says:
yay"

Yes, that is a conversation from msn, and yes, my name was "Houseparty 06- FROM THE INSIDE OUT!!!!!!! And the cry of my heart is to bring You praise." The other participant in the conversation was my good friend Linda. Her name "Its (st) in pindyland" changed depending on the stress we were under due to school homework and assessment. (st) was actually a picture of a storm cloud with lightning. That was worse than the cloud with rain coming out of it and definitely worse than the rainbow picture which would appear when we were cruising along with no looming assessment.

My name comes from a Youth Group camp. No, Houseparty does not stand for a wild party that happens when the parents are away. Definitely not! I stay far away from anything like that! Houseparty 06 was the annual church Youth Group camp in which the Youth went away for a weekend to grow in our faith, have extended times of worship, and do crazy 'fun' activities (I wasn't so much into the crazy activities). The theme for 2006 was "From the inside out" which is also the name of a song by Hillsong. The special guest for the weekend was Brett, the Junior Band leader from our corps (church). He had a real passion for evangelism and knew that our life with God needs to work its way out from the inside. We need to have an ongoing close personal relationship with God in order to effectively witness for Him. We need to know Him so we can tell others what He is like and who He is. Brett also had many hilarious stories. It was a great weekend and clearly it impacted me since I made it my msn name for so long.

So, back in the world of msn and life as a Year 12 student, Linda and I were helping each other prepare for our upcoming Physics test in early 2007. Well, Mum would protest and say, "It's not a test, it's an exam" because a test sounded too little, too insignificant, too simple for senior students. Plus, in Year 12, every assessment exuded a bit of extra pressure because it would contribute to our HSC.

For those of you who don't live in NSW, you may be wondering "what is the HSC?" Well, it is meant to show how much we know by the end of our schooling and stands for "Higher School Certificate", but what it really does is put an immense amount of pressure on all Year 12 students to remember copious amounts of information about mostly irrelevant or obscure topics. I guess it prepares us well for university!

At the end of the year, we are given an HSC mark for each subject and a UAI (now known as an ATAR) which helps universities select students for their courses. The higher your UAI, the more likely you will get into the course you want. It is very mysterious how the marks are calculated but one day our Year 11 Chemistry teacher who was 'in the know' explained it to us. Well, she explained the HSC mark part. The UAI is still a mystery.

Anyway, for all the NSW students who are wondering how it works, here is the secret:

Your HSC mark is broken down into two components: School Mark (50%) and Exam Mark (50%). These two marks are calculated and then added together to give you your HSC mark for each subject. These names are a bit misleading. What really counts for your School Mark is where you rank in your school for each subject and what really counts for your Exam Mark is how you perform in your HSC exam during

October/November. That one exam counts for 50% of your mark!   Whatever you get in your HSC exam equates to 50% of your mark for that subject. You get your School Mark by finding the HSC exam mark that matches your individual rank in your class and then you add the 2 components together to get your HSC mark for that particular subject. Confused yet?

Linda and I would often help each other study … we almost did all the same subjects throughout our senior years. Physics was definitely not one of our favourites, but some of the topics were quite interesting.

My life was busy. As well as studying 12 units for my HSC (you only have to do 10 units), I was also playing in the school Stage Band, having piano lessons from my Nana, tutoring guitar to one student and giving upper-level primary homework help for another student, plus being involved at church with Youth Group, weekly church services and the musical sections.

This was a typical week for me at that time:

Sunday: Wake up and go to church for 'Corps Cadets' (a program that was like Sunday School but for teenagers). Catch up with other people from church during the morning tea. Come home for lunch and work on homework or assignments, or relax if everything was up to date. Then once a month we had a night church service as well and sometimes we had Youth Group Suppers on a Sunday night. I enjoyed the night church services. We would often have a testimony time where anyone could stand up and testify of something God had done in their life recently. It was exciting and encouraging to hear the stories. We even had a group of men that would come to the night church services who were residing at a rehab centre. They would share great stories of God helping them get free of addictions.

Monday: Go to school from 8:12am (Roll Call) until 4:00pm (Extension 1 Maths was after school). Tutor guitar to a student 7pm-8pm. Work on homework and assignments and study for upcoming tests as needed.

Tuesday: Go to school from 8:12am (Roll Call) until 4:00pm (Stage Band rehearsal was after school). 4:30pm-5:30pm Tutor/Homework help for an upper-level Primary student. Work on homework and assignments and study for upcoming tests as needed.

Wednesday: Go to school from 8:12am (Roll Call) until 2:38pm (Normal school finishing time). Piano lesson with Nana. Work on homework and assignments and study for upcoming tests as needed.

Thursday: Go to school from 8:12am (Roll Call) until 4:15pm (Extension 2 Maths was after school). Work on homework and assignments and study for upcoming tests as needed.

Friday: Go to school from 8:12am (Roll Call) until 12pm (early finish because of the Extension subjects I had to stay after school for on other days). Work on homework and assignments and study for upcoming tests as needed. Junior Band rehearsal at church on Friday evening.

Saturday: Try to sleep in. Work on homework and assignments and study for upcoming tests as needed. Relax and have fun. Sometimes we had a Youth Group activity on a Saturday night. Also, I helped out in the worship band at a Divisional church Youth event called "Flayva". This was usually on once a month.

As you can see, it was a busy week. I also had to fit in devotions, practising the piano and trumpet, eating, sleeping, showering, chores and so on, but I was loving life! I was also looking forward to the end of high school. I mostly enjoyed school however I remember feeling the urge that it was time to move on when I was in Year 6 and again when I was in Year 12. Although I was only mid-way through Year 12, there was a definite sense of, I am ready to finish now.

I had no idea that I was going to be finishing up sooner than I thought.

Chapter 2:
Stopped in my tracks

Term 2 had been draining. For English, we had been studying Shakespeare's *King Lear*. English was my weakest subject and I did not enjoy it much until Year 10 when we were given an amazing teacher … Mrs Williams. She was so passionate and knowledgeable about her content. Even though I still did not like doing the work, I never wanted to miss a lesson because it was so good to just listen to her (and very helpful for preparing for our assessments). I am so glad we had her for Year 11 and Year 12 because English is compulsory for the HSC. (For some unknown reason it is the only compulsory subject.)

Anyway, back to *King Lear*. We had been given a homework task of making 'Act Summaries'. This does not sound bad on the surface, but the amount of detail we were required to put into them … oh, it was such an effort! It took weeks! On top of all the other things we were doing, it created a lot of late nights, weary eyes and tenacious patience battling with the formatting on Microsoft Word to get these Act Summaries done up nicely and comprehensively in a table. As well as the Act Summaries, we had to do our assessable item: give an oral presentation on *King Lear*. Ughh… speeches… and Shakespeare! Just get through Monday Week 6, I thought, and then we are on the downhill to the holidays.

I gave the oral presentation and genuinely felt a burden be lifted off. Only four and a bit weeks until the holidays and not many assessments left to go. Such a good feeling!

Week 7 began and on Monday night, as I studied for my 2 Unit Maths test, Mum came upstairs with a choc mud scone from Baker's Delight as a treat for supper. She also encouraged me not to stay up too much longer because I would need a good sleep in order to be fresh for tomorrow. My back was feeling a bit sore, so after a little more study I went to bed and drifted off to sleep.

CLICK. On came the radio, 103.2, and I awoke. It was the morning of Tuesday 5th June, 2007. As I came to my senses, I realised that I didn't feel right. I felt awful. I felt like I had been run over by a bus, as the saying goes.

"I don't think I'll be able to wash my hair this morning", I told Mum.

"I feel so tired! I think I might be getting sick. Can you drive me to school today?"

"Are you able to go to school?" Mum asked.

"I have to go today, Mum. I've got my maths test, and you need a doctor's certificate if you miss out on an HSC assessment. And it's Tuesday … Mr Newton will be mad if I miss Stage Band rehearsal."

After deliberating a bit more with Mum we came up with a compromise … Go to school, but don't stay for Stage Band … and Mum will drive me to school.

As we pulled up to the drop off zone, I got out of the car and almost straight away saw Mr Newton …

I really enjoyed Stage Band and I have hardly ever missed any rehearsals, but recently a few people had been missing them, and given that we were getting very close to our recording session, Mr Newton really did not want anyone missing any rehearsals for any reason whatsoever!

Here goes…

"Hey… Umm…"

Come, on, just say it…

"I'm really sorry but I won't be able to stay for Stage Band this afternoon. I'm not feeling well."

His response wasn't so bad. He did try and talk me into staying, but I had to be honest with him and with myself - based on how I was feeling that was definitely not happening! I think he understood, but he was clearly disappointed.

Well, that's done. Now to get through the maths test!

As the day progressed, I did not feel any better … rather I was struggling to keep my head up in class and all I wanted to do was go to sleep. I nearly did go to sleep during my free ('Senior Study Period'). This was extremely unusual for me as I never sleep during the daytime. Even when I was a baby, I am told that I would rarely sleep more than 20 minutes during the day … Something weird was going on in my body.

Somehow, I did the maths test and I really wanted to make it through the day but at lunchtime Linda told me to go to sick bay. That means I would miss English! But she was adamant, "You need to go to sick bay! I'll take you there now," she said. So, off we went.

It felt so good to lie down. My weary, achy body had been crying out to lie down for hours. I listened to the sick bay lady call Mum. Mum was working but she was able to come and pick me up. When she arrived, I said I would meet her out the front of the school.

That was a bit of a mistake … I nearly fainted a few times making my way to the car!

What was happening to me?

Mum was quite concerned when she picked me up. I was relieved to fall into the car, slink into a reclined seat and rest my heavy head and body that was filled with lethargy, aches and pains.

When we arrived home, I went straight to bed and rested all afternoon and evening, although I did make it a few steps to the lounge upstairs and watched a bit of TV with Mum and my sister, Rachel. Dad was away overseas for work. This was about the first time he had ever gone overseas for work.

After the show finished Rachel helped me up and I felt a bit dizzy. I started making my way to the bathroom to get ready for bed.

THUMP.

I woke up lying on the floor in the doorway of the spare room. Mum and Rachel were standing over me. I had fainted. Onto my sister. Apparently, I was very heavy as a dead weight and she did exceedingly well to get me to the floor without too much of a bang or injury to me or to herself!

Chapter 3:
I'll be back soon

You're not going to school tomorrow!" declared Mum. Whatever hopes I had of getting back to school for Wednesday were dashed. I didn't have to make the decision. My body had made it for me. And Mum confirmed it with her emphatic statement. She was speaking wisely. Clearly, given the fainting episode, I didn't have enough strength.

So, I stayed home Wednesday. And the next day. And the day after that ...

Linda was determined to keep me connected and up to date with everything that was going on at school. She thought, as we did, that I would be back at school any day. Initially, we anticipated I would only miss the Tuesday afternoon. But then when I missed Wednesday as well, surely I would be right for Thursday ...

Thursday 07/06/07 7:48pm
"R u feeling any better? We're all starting to really worry about u... When u didnt come to 4unit I suspected something was amiss.
Not that i wanna make u feel worse, but u missed alot today!
An old chemistry teacher came in for a visit... with news that our lovely photo resides on her desk at work.

What you have been waiting for for so long finally happened! Ok, so it wasnt in physics, it was after school (before 4unit). Standing in the canteen, we were all alarmed as waves of people came pouring out of the school - and then we heard the siren

"Attention, attention, attention..."

No, it wasnt a trial! The firemen were on their way and we were all a little apprehensive by this time. Luckily, Mr Burgis came out with some good (?) news:

*"We've had a false alarm ... The alarm was set off by ... *wait for it**

.... a piece of burnt toast!"

Major lols all round (Elyse to DW: "Miss, we can write about this in our memory stories!").

But who was the perpetrator?

We are still unsure, but one thing was certain: about 5 minutes after the alarm went off, Mr Smith and Mr Aitken were seen sheepishly coming out of the staffroom...

Hope you feel better! Attached are the notes. (We still havent got any further in 3unit).

--Linda"

I was missing out on so much at school! Just to be clear, I'm not a pyromaniac and had definitely NOT been waiting for so long for a fire in the school. I hate the smell of smoke and I would not want any harm to come to the school! I had been waiting so long for a drill. The school had recently invested in a fancy new alarm system and they had tested it one afternoon when we were trying to concentrate hard during Extension 1 Maths. They probably thought no one was still in class as it was after school, but we were! It was very distracting, but it was also very different to the old alarm system and I was keen to see how all the other students would react. I know it's meant to be a serious thing, but it came complete with a recorded voiceover message which, together with the over-the-top alarm noises, sounded rather humourous to all of us at the time!

Also attached to this email from Linda were notes on the lessons from the day. Linda was in all of my classes except for Music, so she provided me with a fairly comprehensive overview of everything that I needed to learn and what homework was required so that I wouldn't fall behind. Linda began this trend that very first Tuesday when I had to go home during the day. And almost every day she would send me an email with the notes from the lessons and any random stories to brighten my day. Of course, I could barely lift my head off the pillow, let alone try to do any school work, but I did plan to catch up when I had more energy again. I am so glad Linda sent those emails, even if I couldn't do much with the notes. It really did give me something to look forward to each day.

The weekend arrived. It was a dark and dreary Saturday morning. Poor Mum had to go and pick Dad up from the airport early that day amidst the thunder and lightning with rain pouring down.

The plane inbound from Norway was coming in for approach, but the conditions were too severe.

Landing aborted.

The plane kicked up a gear and began regaining altitude.

"This is your Captain speaking. We will try one more time to land. If it's not possible we will be diverted to Melbourne or Brisbane."

After circling around, the plane began its descent for a second time.

Landing gear engaged. Altitude decreasing.

Touchdown.

Welcome back, Dad!

I was glad to see Dad. He was concerned for me and was glad to be home. Mum told him not to go away again because drastic things always seem to happen when he is not around! From giant spiders to blackouts and now me getting so sick. Things seem to be better when he is around. Maybe I would get better now?

Later that day I went to the GP. My blood tests showed that I had mild neutropenia, which means I had a virus. We didn't have any treatment for it, but at least I knew medically that there was definitely something going on in my body.

After about a week of not being at school I had a phone call from some of the staff to find out how I was going and let me know they were praying for me to get better. Ever the optimist I said I should be right in another week.

It was so encouraging to know I had prayer support from these trusted adults in my life and to know that I was being missed – not forgotten. Being part of this Christian school was a real blessing – particularly during those long, hard days.

When I was not 'right in another week' I figured that I would surely be back after the holidays...

Chapter 4:
What's going on?

The next few weeks were a blur of doctor visits, fighting off the illness, being exhausted and looking forward to being better.

It must be a bad case of the flu we all thought.

Each morning I woke up hoping to be all better – after all, throughout my life whenever I was not feeling great Dad would always tell me, "Do you know what you need? You need a big sleep!" And thankfully, most nights I slept really well. But I was not improving. Sure, the congestion and a few of the bodily aches eased off, but I just had no energy whatsoever!

By Friday 15th June I was still no better so it was back to the doctor. We could not get into my usual GP, but were able to get an appointment with another one at the same practice. He advised that I was bordering on pneumonia and prescribed Rulide antibiotics. I had a continual lethargy, was unable to concentrate and had an aching back, muscles and joints.

On Monday it was my great grandmother's funeral. It was a cold, windy winter's day and there was no way I could make it to the cemetery and the funeral service, so I went to the cemetery for the burial. It is the first time that someone I knew personally had died. Mum and Dad were helping me stand up and I was coping ok until I saw the coffin being lowered into the ground and my Nana (it was her mother who had died) was crying. The pain of death became real. Death is such an enemy, ripping away those we love from us. I began to appreciate the hope we have as Christians a lot more. We know we will see our loved ones again because of Jesus' gift of eternal life. Though we die, yet we will live again.

The next day we had an appointment with my usual GP. He confirmed that my chest was clear. This was good news as pneumonia would have been affecting my chest. We were given a referral for a specialist, which we booked in for the following Monday (25th June). This specialist physician didn't think there was much wrong with me. "You'll be back to school this time next week," he said.

That did NOT happen!

But what did happen was a prayer meeting. That Tuesday night our church leader, a group of friends from church and some extended family came to my house. I was lying on the couch downstairs and they were sitting all around the room.

Uncle Tim arrived mid-way through the prayer meeting and began to read some Scripture.

James 5:13-16 *"Is anyone among you in trouble? Let them pray. Is anyone happy? Let them sing songs of praise. 14Is anyone among you sick? Let them call the elders of the church to pray over them and anoint them with oil in the name of the LORD. 15And the prayer offered in faith will make the sick person well; the LORD will raise them up. If they have sinned, they will be forgiven. 16Therefore confess your sins to each other and pray for each other so that you may be healed. The prayer of a righteous person is powerful and effective."* (NIV)

"Dana, I need to ask you, is there any sin you can think of that you need to confess?" Uncle Tim asked me gently.

"Umm…" My heart was racing. Definitely not expecting that question, but I guess it is in the Scripture.

"Not that I can think of. I'm sure there are many things I've done wrong in my life, but I can't think of anything specific right now".

"Ok, that's fine. I just needed to ask."

"Julie, do you have some oil?" he asked Mum. Of course, we had olive oil and vegetable oil, but Mum wanted something that smelt nice.

"Here's some rose oil," she said triumphantly.

Uncle Tim walked back over to me.

"I'm going to anoint you with this oil. It's just rose oil – nothing special about it by itself. It says in that passage from James to anoint with oil in the name of the Lord and pray over you."

I felt the cool oil being rubbed on my forehead. I began to relax again. Uncle Tim said a lovely prayer asking for my healing. For some reason I was not convinced it was going to work … I was doubting. I believed God could heal and I believed He would heal me … eventually; but just not right away.

Despite the wonderful time of prayer we shared, the next day I was particularly exhausted. It was like I had gone backwards. I had been slowly improving … I was beginning to stay awake more throughout the daytime and was getting brighter in myself. My head was still very heavy though and I always had to lean it on something.

My GP was rather puzzled with what was going on, as were we! After a while, we realised that the flu-like symptoms had all but gone, yet I still had no energy. So, it MUST be *glandular fever*, right?

Glandular fever is a virus that attacks the body and has similar symptoms to the flu, however, it lingers on for about six weeks (sometimes shorter and sometimes longer) and you can't really do anything while you have it because your body is so weak. To the average person, glandular fever sounds like a nightmare. Who would ever want to be bedridden for six weeks? Who has the time for that these days? How could I possibly miss six weeks' worth of school? And not just any year of schooling, but my final year ... the year of the HSC, packed full of content-heavy lessons in order to get through the overcrowded curriculum in the time frames given and littered with regular pressure-filled assessments which all count towards and heavily impact upon my future ...

No, you definitely don't want to get glandular fever in Year 12.

That is, unless you have already been sick for four weeks and you don't have a clue what is causing this lingering, excessive, all-encompassing fatigue ... Yes, at that point I wanted to have glandular fever! Only two more weeks? That's ok. I can cope with that! I had become sick in Week 7 of Term 2. It was now the end of Term 2 and we had three weeks of holidays coming up. If glandular fever lasts for six weeks, I should be right for the start of Term 3, or very close to it.

As you can imagine, my family were also hoping it was glandular fever. So, the GP had me tested for it ...

The results came back negative.

I did not have glandular fever. My glands were not swollen and whatever virus I had had was gone. Perhaps now I would get better. My GP encouraged me to rebuild my fitness. "Start by walking for five minutes a day," he told me. "You can also try some hydrotherapy and some multivitamins."

But I still was not improving much. It felt like we were back to square one. No one knows what it is or how long it will last for. All we can do is pray that it will go away.

As we kept pressing for answers my GP found one for us. Sort of. He decided it was *post-viral fatigue.* That simply means I had a virus, now I don't have a virus, but I am still sick. Great. What virus had I had? The GP gave us the option of investigating that, but given that it was gone now it really did not matter and I certainly did not have the energy to go to more doctor appointments and have more tests done, especially if there was no real point to it.

I wanted to save up what little energy I had for other things. Like a little bit of exercise to make sure my muscles didn't fade away, praying, reading through the notes Linda was sending me so I was not totally falling behind in my studies, getting back to school as soon as possible, and participating in the Stage Band Recording.

We had been rehearsing for this recording and looking forward to it as a band for many weeks, and although I had missed the last few weeks of term, I was really hopeful that I could at least attend the recording. I really wanted to be able to be part of it so I tried to practice the pieces when I had a bit of energy and made it to one holiday rehearsal on 11th July, but paid for it in exhaustion the following day. I still aimed to get to the recording. It was scheduled for the last weekend of the school holidays: Saturday 21st and Sunday 22nd July, at Trackdown Studios (part of the Fox Studios complex).

The morning of Saturday 21st July I woke up feeling cold. But today was the day, so I read the Word for Today devotional and got dressed, had some breakfast and was driven to Fox Studios. Although most people would think the walk from the car was nothing, it was a very long walk for me in my hindered physical condition. Thankfully upon arriving I was able to have a long sit down and then a long lie down on a couch that was available. I stayed from 11am-1pm and was able to participate in recording six songs.

I had my trusty 'green' pillow with me. This pillow came with me everywhere I went because my head felt so heavy that I struggled to hold it up. Having the pillow meant that I could lean back and rest my head more comfortably on a chair. I thought the pillow was blue, but Mum thought it looked green. I also sat down for the recording, whilst everyone else in the horn section was standing up to play. There was no way I would have had the strength or stamina to stand up and play, so I was very grateful that they repositioned the mic so I could sit down and play the trumpet.

After the recording I had to struggle back to the car via the long walk, and then I rested in the car and the whole remainder of the day when I arrived home.

That night I could not get to sleep until after midnight and then woke at 5am, 6am, 7am and finally got up at 8am. It was not a good sleep. But, the second day of recording was at hand, so I was driven in to Fox Studios again and the day went very much like the day before. On this day we recorded a song that I was meant to play a solo in. That was not possible, so Mr Newton played it instead. That was disappointing, but overall, I knew it was a huge achievement to even get there. We also began the olive leaf extract tonic that afternoon. Eww! It was disgusting! Not the nicest way to end the weekend, but I was still thrilled that I was able to be a part of the recording, despite the immense obstacles.

Chapter 5:
The new normal

How things had changed! From being a busy Year 12 student counting down the days to the end of my schooling, to barely having the strength to get out of bed each day. Completely out of the blue. No warnings. No solutions. Just dealing with it.

My new normal was anything but 'normal'. Apart from medical appointments and the occasional outing to church, school or a family/friend's place (very rare), I would be at home ... in bed, or on the couch. Everything was a huge effort, even the smallest things like trying to sit up in bed, let alone get out of the bed. I was often cold, despite what the weather was doing and even when rugged up inside my bed. My body would ache, particularly my back, neck and stomach. My head felt too heavy for my neck to hold up – it felt as if someone was pushing it backwards. I often felt like I was in a daze. When I wanted to stand up, I had to gradually sit, then wait, then be pulled up by Mum or Dad. I felt really dizzy and my legs could hardly support me – I needed someone to support me walking most of the time. The overwhelming feeling of exhaustion was persistent, with fleeting moments of feeling less drained. The exhaustion is not simply just feeling very tired. No. Rather it is like you have just run a marathon. Your whole body is so worn out that it fails to do the simplest of tasks. Even after a long sleep, it was common to wake up still feeling utterly exhausted. Some nights I would sleep through, but others I would wake multiple times through the night despite being so tired.

Some days I could do a little bit of school work, but other days I could not concentrate enough to do any of it. Some days I could read books, but other days I did not even have the strength to hold the book up while I was lying in bed. Some days I could watch TV (Ready Steady Cook became a favourite) or a DVD, but other days I did not have the ability to concentrate and my head would just ache and be dizzy. Some days I would be able to sit up for a while, but other days I would have to be lying down all the time.

Some days I would be hungry, but other days I lost my appetite. Some days I could chat with Linda and other friends on msn/email, but other days reaching across to my laptop next to my bed was too exhausting.

Some days I could pray, but other days my mind was too tired to think of what to say. Some days I felt like this sickness was overwhelming and fully real, but other days I doubted I was truly sick despite all the symptoms.

But every day my family was there for me. Every day people were praying for me. Every day God was sustaining me physically and mentally. Because of this, I never lost hope. I never got depressed. I never gave up believing I would eventually be healed.

Early on in my sickness, my sister, Rachel (14yrs), began to come into my room every day with a Bible verse that she had selected, typed up, printed out, cut out with crinkly scissors and either coloured in or printed on coloured cardboard. She would read it out to me and then stick it somewhere in my room – on my corkboard at the foot of my bed, on my wardrobe doors to the right of my bed, on my bookshelf between the doorway and the wardrobe, on my chest of drawers to the left of my bed, along the edge of the shelf above my desk in the corner of my room …

As the days passed by, I became literally surrounded by the Word of God … the promises of God … My wonderful, compassionate, kind-hearted sister in this simple act of obeying the prompting of the Holy Spirit did something profoundly powerful for me. This was special. This was important. This helped lift me up. I praise God for her faithfulness! I was so blessed in this!

One day she came in with 1 Peter 5:7 *"casting all your care upon Him, for He cares for you."* This one really stood out. I kept coming back to it over and over again. We don't need to carry our burdens. God invites us to hand them over to Him. He will carry them for us. And He will carry us too. He really will.

Every day that I had ventured downstairs my Dad would help me back upstairs in the evening. Sometimes he would carry me down the stairs just so I was not stuck upstairs all day. Sometimes he would also carry me back up.

There were 15 stairs. 15 is a lot. 15 is distressing. 15 seems insurmountable. Dad knew this. So, to him there were only 2 stairs. The one we were doing and the next one. "One," he would say as we climbed the first step. "One," he would say as we climbed the second step. "One," he would say as we climbed the third step, and the fourth step, all the way to the fourteenth step. Then, as we climbed the final, fifteenth step, he would joyfully exclaim "Two!" We had very slowly, yet successfully, made it up the stairs.

Every day that I was sick Mum was there comforting me, taking me to and from medical appointments, praying for me, praying with me, and encouraging me to exercise. We had a 10-metre swimming pool in our backyard and Mum suggested that I walk around it for my initial walks. It was important to get out into the fresh air and sunshine (if there was any). So, I tried one lap around the pool and gradually built up to five laps. It was barely what you could call walking. It was more of a shuffle or plodding one foot in front of the other. Walking five laps was hard! As I slowly inched my way around the pool, in which I used to swim 100 laps, I focused on remembering what lap I was up to and looked forward to getting back inside to lie down. But Mum was there to cheer me on and help me not give up.

As I continued day by day, God highlighted the story of the Israelites in the wilderness to me. It was coming alive – just as they could only take manna enough for one day, and had to trust God that He would provide manna again the next morning, I had to trust God to provide strength for one day, and then trust He would provide strength again the next morning (see Exodus 16).

Many days I would also be encouraged by family and friends who had sent me Get Well cards, Thinking of You cards, flowers, chocolates, and so on. Linda organised a massive card, which she made herself with an A3 piece of cardboard. She invited many of my peers at school and my teachers past or present to write on the card. On Friday 22nd June, Rachel delivered the card home to me. It was so lovely to receive! So many wonderful messages (and a few silly ones too – thanks to the teenage boys!).

Around the end of September, Rach organised a book with numerous encouraging messages and prayers from family, friends and teachers both from school and from church. Again, I am so thankful for my sister's willingness to go the extra mile and make sure I knew I was cared for and loved. This support was holding me up and reminding me that though I was mostly stuck at home, I was not forgotten. Dad wrote a message in this book which touched me deeply and encouraged me in what I was believing for... *you show us your smile all the time even though you must be asking why me at times! We know God will show us all in His time why, and heal you fully."*

One day, healing will come.

About six weeks into the sickness, I found a small bit of energy to pick up my pen and make a journal entry...

"Dear Jesus, I haven't journaled really since I got sick – 6 weeks and 1-2 days ago. It's been hard, relaxing, comforting, humbling, testing, and a lot of other things too. I know You've been with me every step of the way. I thank You for Your peace and assurance that my life is in Your hands! Promises from Your Word have helped a lot – I know You have a plan and purpose for my life from Jeremiah 29:11 and in Jeremiah 30:17a I see now... ""I will bring back your health, and heal your injuries," says the LORD." (NCV) What a promise for such a time as this! Thank You for leading me to this reminder – You constantly remind me of Your healing power... through Your Word – Jesus healed many and through His name so many are healed! And even today's verse! And through other people = cards, words of encouragement, messages etc. Thank You for all of that – keeping me positive..."

"I'm learning to trust You more especially with my future – can't control sickness -> can't control UAI -> can't control course at Uni -> can't control job. But You can control and are in control and I've got to trust You and I know that I will still have some control in these things but I hand over the control to You – lead me Lord I will follow! May I listen to Your leading and trust You more!"

Chapter 6:
Searching for answers

The day after the Stage Band recording was the first day of Term 3. The school had organised for me to meet with the Head Teacher of Teaching and Learning (Mr CJ), the Principal (Dr B), and the Deputy Principal (Mr M). We needed to figure out a plan moving forward.

I was quite worn out from the weekend's efforts, but I knew I had to come along to this meeting. It would be nice to see my friends afterwards as well. I was anxious about what I might find out or what I might have to do.

… Would I need to repeat Year 12?

… Would I need to come back to school even if I was not 100%?

… Would I need to continue to try and do all my assessments, even the ones I had missed already?

Mum prayed with me and helped to reassure me that this was going to be a good thing to have the meeting. We will at least have a plan to work with.

I sat down in the room, pillow and all, and still felt nervous. I did not really know Mr CJ as he was a new staff member. The principal was also fairly new in his role. Mr CJ explained that I needed to make sure I had done at least 50% worth of my school-based assessment for each subject. Given my condition, they did not want to force me to try and complete anything beyond that. 50% would be sufficient to estimate the rest of my marks.

Wow! This was great news! I did not need to repeat Year 12. This was a massive relief.

I did have some work to do though. I had completed enough assessment for Advanced English and Physics, but between 40% and 45% for Extension 1 Mathematics, Ext 2 Mathematics and Music 1.

For Chemistry I had officially completed 30%, but there was an assessment due about a week after I fell ill which would take me above the 50% threshold. I brought this with me to the meeting. Although I had been stuck at home fighting off this worse than flu-like illness, school continued and I knew that I would need to submit my Chemistry Assessment. It was a First-Hand Investigation on "Separating a Mixture of Organic Materials in Pigments". In ordinary language that means discovering the pigments in a leaf. I had to conduct my own experiment at home and write a full scientific report on it, complete with Aim, Materials, Method, Results, Discussion, Conclusion. I hadn't finished it when I got sick as there was still a week left to complete it. Thankfully I had already done the experiment and begun to write up the report. However, despite trying to finish it off, I could not. I had to submit it incomplete. I felt terrible as I always wanted to complete my assessments to the best of my ability, but I just had to realise that handing in something almost finished was better than handing in nothing. My Chemistry teacher was very understanding and encouraged me that what I had done was very good.

Over the next few days, I found out that I needed to attempt part of the Trial Exam for Extension 1 and Extension 2 Mathematics. I was given permission to do this from home under Mum's supervision at a time when I had some energy. This was very kind. I had no idea how I would be able to do the exams, but I knew that by being able to do them at home I could at least lie down when I needed to and not use up all my energy in getting to school.

For Music 1, I was asked to play one of my pieces during the Music Trial Exam, which was on Wednesday 1st August at school.

As for the HSC, we would see how I was going when that was closer, but I would definitely be eligible for misadventure forms. This means I would get special consideration and my school ranks would give the examiners a good indication of what I was capable of pre-illness. They would then adjust my exam mark accordingly.

As we finished up in the meeting I was feeling more at ease, but still anxious about how it would all play out. I enjoyed visiting my maths class briefly before we went back home and I had a big rest.

That afternoon I went to hydrotherapy. This is exercise in a shallow swimming pool. I had begun this just one week earlier after my GP had suggested it. The good news was the pool was indoors (no sunscreen required) and heated (great for the cooler days!). The bad news was that all the other patients were old people doing rehabilitation therapy after hip or knee replacements and the like. I felt very out of place. As we walked up and down the pool, they were strides ahead of me. I felt rather discouraged. Although, at least I did manage to swim faster than they did. We also had to lean on a pool noodle and cycle our legs, and hold a short pool noodle underneath the water and move it around to build up the arm muscles as well. It was a big workout for my weakened muscles and my exhausted body. I needed a long rest after every session – it really took what little energy there was out of me.

The next day was Mum's birthday. Dad woke me up and we gave Mum some gifts before he went to work. Later on,

Mum drove me to her parents' house and we did a 500-metre walk. It took me 16 minutes and 50 seconds! At least I was walking, but oh how different things were!

I opened my eyes and could barely see that Mum and Nana were entering my room. I tried to sit up. My body would not budge. I tried to say something. My words would not come out. In a bit of a panic, I tried again.
Nothing.
Eyes closed.
I opened my eyes and saw Mum and Nana entering my room again. I tried to say hello, but could not. I tried to get up, but my body would not cooperate. I felt so dizzy.
Eyes closed.
I opened my eyes and there they were. Mum and Nana at the end of my bed. Why couldn't I move or talk?
What is going on?
Eyes closed.
I opened my eyes. They were gone. I took a while to take all my surroundings in. I was in bed. Nana had not been there at all, neither had Mum. I had just had some hallucinations. They seemed so real. I began to calm down as I realised that I could move and talk and what I had thought was real, actually did not happen.

I woke up and stared at the clock radio by my bed. 3:00am. It had been hard to get to sleep last night.
Why am I awake? This is not time to get up! Back to sleep.
I stirred again. To my disappointment, it was still very dark. 4:00am.

Sigh … back to sleep.

I rubbed my tired eyes … 5am. It is not time to wake up yet!

Again, I woke up … 6am. This makes no sense. I am so tired, but my body will not stay asleep. I'll try again.

7am.

8am. I am so tired!

9:10am. It's Monday 30th July. I am going for a school visit today. I better get up.

After a few stretching exercises, breakfast and dressing in my school uniform, Mum drove me to school in time for recess. It was nice to get out and see my friends, but the walking around was exhausting. The main point of the visit was to touch base with my teachers. My Biblical Studies and Leadership teacher, Mr Bell, told me that he had had chronic fatigue for six years, and here he was working as a teacher now. There was some hope. My Physics and Chemistry teacher, Mr Aitken, told me to watch a show on the ABC on Friday, "As it is in heaven". He also said my Chemistry assessment was ok. Mrs Williams said "Don't worry about English, we can catch up in one day". Now that's optimism! My Maths teacher, Mr Stanley, wanted an update about whether or not I was doing my HSC.

I slumped into the car. I was done. Time for a big rest and hopefully some better sleep.

That night I was looking forward to a good sleep.

I opened my eyes to see the darkened room … dare I look at the clock?

4am.

Oh no!

I woke again at 5am, 6am, 7am and 8:47am. Finally, at 9:53am I forced myself up and out of bed for some breakfast. Hydrotherapy was on this morning.

I really hope this waking up through the night cycle does not continue!

After one of our GP appointments, we left with a prescription for some tablets that might help. Mum went to the pharmacy and brought them home to me. I was hesitant. I didn't think that this was the answer we were looking for. I had an uneasy feeling about it.

Inside the box was a pamphlet listing all the possible side effects ... *depression* ...

My stomach churned.

How could this be something helpful with all those side effects? And especially with depression listed as one of them?

No. This is not for me.

"Sorry Mum, I can't take these ... I don't feel that it's the right thing to do. It's got depression as a side effect! ... I'm keeping positive and I know God will heal me sometime. I don't want to let the enemy have any chance of taking me into depression."

I handed the box back to Mum.

She accepted my decision and the entire box of tablets ended up in the bin.

As I spent so much time lying down, it was important to have a bit more guidance on what exercises I could do. We were told to try an exercise physiologist. I had never heard of such a thing, and was not all that keen for more medical appointments, but we may as well give it a go.

Mum drove us there and we were blessed to find a park right out the front. Thank You, Lord. We got out and walked to the door. Then I stared. It was a staircase. Oh no, I thought. This is another reason not to come here.

Mum helped me get up the stairs and we went in to the consultation room. The exercise physiologist was a young man, full of energy. His chair was a large blue exercise ball, which he sat on with ease. That cannot be comfortable, I thought. That would require a lot of effort too! He then encouraged me that he had recovered from having chronic fatigue himself.

Around this time, we were thinking that my mystery illness, given the underwhelming label "post-viral fatigue", would turn into chronic fatigue syndrome. What is that? Basically, the same as post-viral fatigue, except you need to have been excessively tired for at least six months before you can be diagnosed with it. Thrilling. I did not like the sound of that, but given the very little improvements and the one step forward, two steps back halting of progress I was experiencing, I had come to expect that I would be heading that way.

The exercise physiologist gave me an exercise regime to follow. The exercises were mostly stretches which I needed to do repeatedly in sets of five, twice a day if possible. He also told me how to build up my walks so that they would be longer and not as exhausting for me. "Do 10 seconds fast walking, 5 seconds slow walking, then repeat for your whole walk." "The slow walk is a recovery time". "Once you can do this comfortably, build up to 20 seconds fast, 10 seconds slow, 30 seconds fast, 15 seconds slow, 1 minute fast, 30 seconds slow, and so on."

Mum wanted to make my walks enjoyable so she began to take me to a quiet street which ended with a launching ramp overlooking the Georges River. It was a lovely spot when the sun was shining and the breeze was minimal. It was definitely an upgrade from walking laps around the pool.

With this new method of fast, slow, fast, slow, we also began to be more consistent in our walks. No matter the conditions - rain, wind or sun, we were out there walking. Sometimes Dad would come with us as well. He was not very good at walking slowly. He would often confuse my 'fast' for the slow bit. He wasn't far wrong. My 'fast' was very slow compared to normal. Mum wrote in her journal that an 87-year-old lady walked faster than me early on in my illness.

Tuesday 11th of September. I woke at 2:45am. I had been struggling to get to sleep the last few nights, but once I got to sleep, I had been sleeping through the nights fairly well. I did not want to go back to multiple night wakings again!

I soon managed to fall asleep again but woke up fairly early when Rachel was quietly placing a Bible verse on my door. I could not get back to sleep after that.

Eventually I willed myself out of bed. It was time for another school visit. The exercise physiologist had added some relaxation techniques to my exercise regime – this involved simply lying on a pool noodle on the floor for a few minutes and then lying flat on the floor for a few minutes. Unusual, but it actually felt so good to lie flat on the floor after lying with the pool noodle underneath my back! Anyway, I had 20 minutes of 'relaxation' before showering, having breakfast and heading off to school. Showering always took a lot out of me. Maybe I should have done the relaxation after the shower.

I spent about an hour and a half at school, attending Music and English. Afterwards I was happy, but exhausted and I let out a big sigh...

"Mum, I just want to get better now."

The next day we continued on with our mission of searching for answers in the hope that I would find a way to get better. We had an appointment with another specialist. This one specialised in dealing with patients who had chronic fatigue. Although it had not been six months, we did not want to wait that long before seeing him. I had the same ongoing symptoms that someone with chronic fatigue had, the only difference being mine had been ongoing for a shorter period of time.

"You will need to have a Glucose Tolerance Test, and a Food Allergy Test as well. I recommend a dose of Vitamin B12 and some dietary changes."

You would think that I would be happy to have some direction and more investigation into what could be causing my symptoms, but this doctor was cold-hearted, rude and discouraging.

He handed us a piece of paper that explained the Glucose Tolerance Test. It was to be a four-hour test in which blood was taken every half an hour. I never liked blood tests. The results would show which type of hypoglycaemia or hyperglycaemia I had. The results left no room to not have either. I was puzzled as to which category would be best to be in. I thought they all sounded abnormal. Where was the normal category?

"The Vitamin B12 is an injection."

I hate needles. I thought vitamin supplements were a tablet. I had been taking a multi-vitamin for weeks now. This was not part of the plan. I was feeling very uneasy with this doctor.

"Which arm do you want to put it in?" I asked nervously and politely.

"Your arm, not mine," he joked.

That was not funny.

After jabbing me with the needle I just wanted to go home, but I kept putting on a brave face.

"Now, I want you to try cutting out some foods. Limit red meat to once a week. Cut out sugar, yeast, citrus, tomatoes..."

Mum's face was looking concerned. I could almost read her thoughts... what are we going to eat!?

"Well, at least I don't like tomatoes." I said, trying to think of a positive.

"You know that tomatoes are in lots of things, don't you? So that means no tomato sauce, no pasta because it's in pasta sauce, no pizza because it's in pizza sauce..." he rebutted in a tone that made me feel reprimanded for daring to find a hint of optimism.

It was yet another abrupt, insensitive response. I felt like crying. Can we go home now? I couldn't wait to get back in the car.

Back home Mum saw me lying on the couch. I was working hard at holding back the tears. Mum saw a tear rolling down my cheek.

"My eyes are just watery." I said, trying to convince myself. But that was like a trigger releasing a build-up of emotions. I started sobbing. It really was so hard. A hard, hard 14 weeks.

Mum came over and comforted me. She was being strong for me. I know this illness was so hard on our whole family. Unbeknown to me, behind the scenes, trying not to in front of me, Mum had already cried many tears for me.

Chapter 7:
Not the tests I was expecting in Year 12

The following Monday I had to go to Pitt Street for my Cytotoxic Food Allergy test. Just to make it there would be pushing myself to the limit. Then once there, it involved taking a lot of blood.

I woke up feeling unrefreshed. I was not allowed to eat any breakfast. We made our way into the city and found the testing centre. They drew the blood from my right arm. It was not a pleasant experience. My arm was very sore afterwards. My left wrist was also aching and my neck was sore.

That afternoon I was exhausted. There was no walk that day.

My arm then ached the next few days after this blood test. I was becoming quite anxious about the Glucose Tolerance Test which I would be having on Thursday. How could I possibly get through nine blood tests in one day? My arm was still sore from the one blood test on Monday...

On Wednesday night I was so exhausted that I crawled up the stairs. Dad was out at church band practice so he wasn't there to carry me up. Although I was so very tired, I couldn't get to sleep until 1am.

On Thursday morning I woke up with a bleeding nose at 7:10am. Given that I needed to fast 12 hours before the Glucose Tolerance Test, I was not allowed any breakfast. I was feeling uneasy about what was ahead of me that morning. Then Rachel gave me such a beautiful letter encouraging me about what I had to face that day.

"I know at times we may struggle with situations that we may be faced with, but just know and remember one important thing: GOD is in control. He is with you always and he never leaves you." … "You are a very special sister and I want you to know that I am here for you. Although I may not be sitting with you at the surgery today, but just know that I will be standing with you through prayer and thoughts."

That definitely helped me to feel a bit better. Mum also prayed with me. She had to go to work but Dad was able to take me to the test. When I got there, Dad prayed with me.

That was a very special moment.

The young pathologist assigned to me came and prepared my arm for the first extraction. This was going to be the largest volume of blood and required two needles. Usually I would have been anxious, but I truly felt the peace of God wash over me. The blood was drawn and I was not sore. Two needles down, seven to go.

Before the next blood extraction, I needed to drink a very sweet drink which tasted like lime cordial. It was bright green. More blood was then taken every half an hour for four hours. The holes from each needle were lined up in a row across the inside of my arms. Six on the left arm and three on the right, along with the hole from Monday's blood test on my right arm. Dad prayed with me before each blood test and I literally felt the peace of God come over me. It also barely hurt at all. God was surely with me. He gave me a very proficient practitioner to do the tests and protected me during the whole process. Dad was also by my side the whole time. In between each test I would rest on a long thin medical mattress with Dad sitting next to me, comforting me and just being there. I will always remember God's answer to our prayers that day.

The dietary changes brought about some interesting experimentation. Mum did not want me to miss out on enjoying my food, so she put in a concerted effort into finding some nice alternatives to accommodate the new restrictions.

No dairy was a big challenge. Previously I had milk on my Weetbix every morning and would often have cheese on toast, cheese as a topping on spaghetti bolognaise, cheese and biscuits as a snack, and occasionally pizza or nachos as a meal. I would also enjoy yoghurt with some fruit as a dessert. Plus, dairy was in many other food products too.

My friend, Linda, was off dairy and she would have goat cheese and goat milk. I had tried goat cheese while at her house and I knew I did not enjoy it. So, Mum decided we should try sheep yoghurt.

One night we had just finished our first course and Dad left the table. He went down the hallway to the study. Meanwhile, Mum began to dish up the dessert. She chopped up some fruit and topped it with the new sheep yoghurt. None of us had tried it before. I was hoping it would be just like 'normal' (dairy) yoghurt.

The bowl was placed in front of me. I stared at it. Mum and Rachel stared at theirs also. Almost simultaneously we placed our spoons in the bowls and scooped up some of the sheep yoghurt. As the smooth, cold substance touched my tongue, the glands at the back of my mouth made their presence known!

You should have seen our faces!

Yuck!

It was so sour. None of us wanted a second bite, that's for sure!

After we each expressed our disgust, we peered over at the empty seat which had a full bowl sitting there ready for Dad to come back and have. We decided to not influence his experience of the sheep yoghurt, but were 99% sure he would not like it either.

He came back and sat down. We tried not to make eye-contact. We all concentrated on keeping straight faces, not giving anything away.

He took a big spoonful and placed it in his mouth.

"That's off!!" he exclaimed.

We all enjoyed a good laugh.

"It's not off. It's sheep yoghurt," we explained.

"Well, I think it's off sheep yoghurt. There's something wrong with it!"

Ahh. Needless to say, we crossed that one off the list as 'never to be tried again'.

Another food conundrum was the 'red meat once a week' restriction. Previously Mum would often cook us meals that contained red meat. Lamb chops in the fry pan, lamb supreme chops as a casserole, beef casserole, spaghetti bolognaise with beef mince, rissoles with beef mince, meatloaf with beef mince, shepherd's pie with beef mince, beef sausages in the oven, Roast Beef, Roast Lamb, and Dad would cook us steak or beef sausages on the BBQ. Cut all those meals out and add on the fact that I don't like fish, and we ended up having a lot of chicken!

At first, I didn't mind. I enjoy chicken. Chicken is good. Chicken can be cooked in a variety of ways to create many different meals. However, we did get a bit bored of chicken, chicken and more chicken. Mum thought we were eating so much chicken that we would all look like chickens!

The worst experience we had was the chicken sausages. We had been missing the beef sausages and when Mum discovered that there was such a thing as chicken sausages, she thought that would be a nice change up from the other chicken meals.

Unfortunately, she was wrong. It is hard to describe exactly what they were like, but perhaps if you imagine chicken feet, chicken gristle, chicken bones, chicken fat and a little bit of chicken flesh blended together with half a salt and pepper shaker worth of salt and wrapped in a thick plastic-like film, you might be getting close. They were awful!

Another item to add to the 'never to be tried again' list!

One final memorable moment with the new diet was Mum's egg and bacon pie – a much loved recipe of Nana's. As I usually would have had Weetbix with milk and brown sugar for breakfast and I was not allowed milk or sugar, and I didn't want to just eat a dry Weetbix, I had to have something else. We found a yeast free lavash bread that I could have with some peanut butter (no vegemite due to its yeast content). However, Mum wanted to do something special for me and so she cooked up an egg and bacon pie (without pastry).

I was lying in bed still and she brought breakfast upstairs to me.

"What is it?", I inquired. The smell had given a little bit away already.

"Egg and bacon pie", Mum explained.

I looked at it and burst out laughing. It was as if the eggs were looking up at me. Baked eggs and bacon with a little bit of onion. It sounded like a nice idea and I thought it would taste nice, but it did make me laugh looking at it.

"Thanks Mum. The eggs," I tried to explain through the laughter, "it's like they are looking up at me!"

When I went to eat it though they were hardened and a bit jelly like. Not all that enjoyable unfortunately.

It was the thought that counted!

Chapter 8:
UAC and graduation

Towards the end of schooling most students apply for university. In NSW the process was to apply online via UAC, the University Admissions Centre. We were advised to study the UAC guide which listed all the previous year's UAI (University Admissions Index) cut-offs for each course at several universities. This would help us know what courses were within our reach based on what marks we were expecting to achieve.

I didn't know what I wanted to do after school. In Year 10 for my work experience I couldn't decide what to explore so I went to three different workplaces: Radiology, Paediatrics, and Macquarie Bank. Before and after the work experience, I didn't think I would end up in any of those workplaces. It was a good experience and they were all interesting … although I was a little bored at the radiology practice. When I found out that new grads had to spend six months on each piece of equipment when they first started out, I thought that would be very monotonous and decided to cross that one off my list. I am sure it would become more interesting if I understood how to interpret the results of the x-rays, CT scans, ultrasounds, angiograms, and MRIs. Anyway, I decided it was not for me.

Now that I was in Year 12, I still did not know what I wanted to do.   All I knew was that I was interested in the medical field, but did not want to do anything that required administering needles or performing surgery. That cuts out a lot of options.

Mum walked into my room one day and I was lying in bed contemplating all the options.

I looked up at her and said, "Mum, I think I want to be a physio."

It made sense to me. It was in the medical field. I had been to physios for my dislocated knee previously and I thought they had a pretty interesting job. It wouldn't get boring because they always had new patients with new conditions. There was a lot to learn about the body with muscles, tendons, ligaments, skeletal structure. I would be helping people … and to my knowledge, they did not have to give needles.

Mum looked down at me and gently pointed out, "Oh honey, you need to have a lot of energy for that. All the massaging. It's very physically demanding."

"That's ok. I'll be better by then, Mum."

I had faith that God would heal me. Even though the sickness was dragging on, I just had this unwavering belief that one day, and one day not too far away, I would be healed.

A little later on I was lying in bed staring at my guitar (which was actually Uncle Mark's but he said I could have it until he moved back to Australia). It was just at the end of my bed on a little stand right by the wall. How I missed playing it. I just wanted to be able to hold it and strum away, singing worship songs to the Lord like I used to. I missed the piano too.

Suddenly, I had another idea.

I could be a music teacher. I like school and I like music and I like to teach people things. I already teach guitar and know how to play a few instruments. Most students like music and I have always had fun playing in school bands and usually enjoyed singing in the choirs.

When I told Mum my new idea, she was a little more on board but also thought it would be very demanding. Part-time work would be an option though. School holidays would be helpful for resting and in the way off future Mum said it would be a great career to have as a Mum because it had a good reputation for providing generous maternity leave, and the school hours and school holidays would make it easier to look after your own kids.

On Saturday 22nd September I put in my UAC application. I decided to put in both options because I still thought being a physio would be good. I applied for five courses as the Music Education and Physio courses were available at multiple universities.

Well... it's done. Now I just need to get through the HSC and see what happens.

The following week was officially my last week of school (though I had not been at school properly since the start of June). On Thursday 27th September I went for a visit so that I could watch the Informal (Muck-Up) Assembly. This was a light-hearted assembly that Year 12 were allowed to run completely on their own, so long as everything was pre-approved by the teachers. There were lots of funny moments, but the highlight for me was the surname story. Everyone's surname from Year 12 was cleverly crafted into a story. It was fun to see how they all came together. Mine was very easy to fit... 'Townsend' not surprisingly became the 'town's end'. Sitting off to the side of the hall I felt a bit out of it, but when I saw my name in the story, I felt I was a little bit part of things again.

The next day was the final day for the class of 2007. It had finally arrived. I was still very sick, but I was able to make it to school for the morning. The Formal Assembly began at 9am.

I entered the hall, which was really a gymnasium with an indoor basketball court, and took my seat next to Mum and Dad along the side near the entrance. Propped up with the pillow I rested my head and looked around.

"Please stand for the Official Party and the singing of the National Anthem", I relished the familiar words. It had been a while since I had heard that phrase.

This was it. My last assembly at school.

Speeches were made and names were called.

"Dana Townsend"

I gingerly made my way to the platform. Just two steps. It really was just two steps, unlike at home with the 15 stairs which Dad pretended were only two.

Once I had navigated the steps, I turned my attention to the staff on the platform. Their tender facial expressions welcomed me as I reached out to receive a book from the first in line, Mrs Gaskell. I moved across towards the principal and he extended his hand towards me for a gentle handshake and a word of encouragement. Next was my homegroup teacher, Mr Power. Every morning (if I was not running late due to traffic) from Year 7 through to Year 12 we started the day as a group and spent extra time together during Homegroup sessions. He shook my hand and gave me a warm smile. Finally, the Year 12 Year Advisor, Mr Smith, shook my hand and then I ever so carefully and slowly made my way to the other side of the room and found a seat. The school community gave me a lovely applause. I was thankful to have made it through that profound moment.

Next was a special morning tea for the Year 12's, staff, parents and siblings. I enjoyed catching up with my friends and teachers. Rachel was so attentive to my needs and was supporting me, getting things for me and taking lots of photos. A blessed morning indeed.

The rest of Year 12 then headed off for the Year 12 picnic, but I went home to rest.

Chapter 9:
HSC

The moment had finally come. The HSC was here. It was such a huge mountain looming on the distant horizon for so long. Actually, way back in primary school it seemed so distant that I was almost convinced that Jesus would come back before I finished Year 12! I suppose this had an element of truth to it. I didn't *really* get to finish Year 12.

Yet, my HSC moment had arrived. Years of preparation, countless hours of study, copious lectures from teachers about how important these exams were to be … and now, after ALL that … I was not even able to scale the mountain … I was not able to sit my exams. It was such an anti-climax! I felt ripped off. I was in this extremely strange position of emotions in which I was right there in the moment vicariously feeling the stress my peers were going through, but at the same time feeling guilty that I was lying down on the couch at home and not being there with them. I knew there was no way I could sit the exams with my fatigue and brain fog as well as all the work I had missed since getting sick, so there was an element of gratitude and relief. Yet, I just felt like I was 'letting the team down' by not doing my HSC exams. What could I do?

I discovered an online community called "Bored of Studies". This was a forum which senior students used to help one another with projects, exams, study and de-stressing. The title was a clever re-imagination of the official department in charge of NSW education called "Board of Studies". I began to be an active member on the site, offering as much help as I could to fellow students. I also spent time praying for my friends as they did their exams, and did what I could to help them with their study. So, I did not feel totally useless and out of it, but it was certainly a weird mix of emotions.

Part of the requirements of the Board of Studies for my HSC misadventure forms was that I needed independent medical evidence as to why I was unfit to sit my exams – given on the day of each of my scheduled exams! With eight exams spread over seven different days this was quite a mission! It seemed like such an illogical thing for me to do when I was so exhausted still. I wanted to put my energy into getting better, not sitting in doctor waiting rooms and sitting through appointments because I had to get a medical certificate AGAIN! But it's what we had to do, so we did it! Mum organised it amazingly. She is a wonderful administrator.

My GP summarised how I was during those days *"extreme lethargy and weakness... unable to concentrate for longer than 10-15 minutes. Any attempt of physical activity for longer than 30 minutes leaves her feeling extremely exhausted and needs to sleep for extended periods to recover ... has been particularly weak, fatigued and dizzy"*.

Mum also managed to give me some variety for these appointments as we went to the GP, the exercise physiologist and a nutritionist.

The nutritionist was a breath of fresh air for us all. I was a little apprehensive going to another person who was going to analyse my diet and potentially give me even less to eat, but we had heard good things about this lady. To our delight, what we were suspecting was true – she was lovely, understanding, encouraging and made a lot of sense. She asked me if I enjoyed taking the olive leaf extract and if I felt better when I had taken it. No and no. She told me she would not be taking something that she did not like if it was not producing any improvements. She said that it seemed the diet I had been put on was not giving the intended results, so it would be better to go back to eating more of the things I enjoyed, but still keeping a focus on making it healthy. I was so relieved. Hooray!!

With the HSC over and the newfound freedom with my diet things were beginning to look up.

Chapter 10:
Auditioning

Part of the requirements for the Music Education degree I had applied for through UAC was to do a live practical audition at the university ...

Audition? ... My stomach churned nervously ... Every year since I was in Year 3, I had to do a piano exam and they were always a nerve-wrecking experience!   After completing Grade 8 Piano in Year 11 I had hoped the only exams I would be doing were the HSC Music 1 practicals. Even so, I was studying enough subjects that I had 12 units and you only need 10 units for the HSC, so the 2 units of Music 1 may not even count towards my HSC. That took a lot of pressure off.

But a university audition ... after not being able to practice for months, not being able to concentrate much, struggling to sit up without my head resting on a pillow ... was it even possible? On top of that, the travel alone would take a lot out of me ... the university was a good 25-minute drive away if there was no traffic. In Sydney there is almost always traffic and the trip could easily take up to an hour in peak times.

We discovered that a pre-recorded audition may be an option. Typically, these were used for students applying from remote regional areas, interstate or internationally. *"Other applicants must apply in writing to submit a tape audition and include a suitable reason,"* stated the website. Mum rang the university and explained my situation and requested that I submit a pre-recorded audition rather than travelling into the university for a live in-person audition.   We were given a verbal 'ok' but we still needed to apply online. Mum got on to it and swiftly prepared a document outlining why I could not attend a live audition. It was the 7th October. If approved, our deadline to submit the audition was 17th November.

Soon enough our request was approved and we began figuring out what pieces of music I would need to perform. The requirements were to include lots of supporting documentation, *"Two contrasting works"* and *"A short song to be sung unaccompanied"*.

Hmmm. A short song. I don't mind singing with a choir, but I am not that excited about singing a solo. The majority of songs I knew were church songs too. Not sure how that would go down at a secular university ...   I am all for witnessing, but I don't think this would be the best way to do it.

Mum came to the rescue again ... "How about "The Long and Winding Road"? That's what the last few months have felt like!"

I sighed ... and smiled. "That's true", I agreed.

This was a song by The Beatles.   Mum and Dad had a recording of someone famous singing it so I kind of knew it ...

"Ok" ... "Let's try that one".

This was the only song we would need to record because I already had the *"Two contrasting works"* recorded from earlier in the year. We had one that was recorded in August for my final Music assessment at school. Mum sourced the other recording from my half yearly exams before I got sick, from Mr Newton. Thankfully he had recorded our assessable performances at school.

On 12th November we had the audition material all ready to go, complete with a declaration, covering letter, references and music certificates, Year 12 Half Yearly HSC

Report, Awards and Participation certificates, Medical Certificates, CD and DVD. Wow. I signed it and we sent it in.

Now ... we wait.

I was so thankful that Mum could organise it all for me and help me learn the song. I know God was helping us through too. Things were falling into place. Maybe I *would* be able to study at university next year ...

Chapter 11:
Formally finished

One of the big end of school events that students get to enjoy (or endure) is the Year 12 formal. Whilst it is definitely not as prestigious as the American version, 'The Prom', it is something that a lot of students, particularly females, get quite excited about. I am not one of those students who was 'quite excited'. I liked the idea of spending time with friends and having a graduation dinner, but I was not really into the whole build-up with finding the dress and so on … I also wanted nothing to do with any after parties and was dreading the thought of what might go on there. Hopefully everyone would be sensible and stay safe.

I was not sure if I would be able to go to the formal anyway with my illness, especially given it would be a late night, but Mum was very keen for me not to miss out on such a special event. The school invited all the parents along so that was really the reason I was able to still go. With Mum and Dad there to support me and take me home when I couldn't last any longer, it was something achievable for me to aim at.

Now that it was established that I could go to the formal, Mum began her mission of finding a dress for me. One day she brought home two possible options for me to try.

First one … no good.

Second one … Mum was really hopeful … but alas, it was no good as well.

Off she went to return the rejected dresses to the shops.

After that she decided I needed to try the dresses on at the shops … so somehow, we made it to the shops and there I was, formal dress shopping with Mum.

Somehow, we found a dress. Mum was pleased I had something nice to wear. I was relieved we did not need to do any more shopping.

Mum wanted to make the night something special for me. She organised our family hair dresser to straighten my hair the day before the big event. She invited my cousin, Lacey, around on the afternoon of the formal to help me get ready.

Finally, it was time to go. It was a bit of a relief to get in the car and be able to rest on the way there. The venue was Dockside, Darling Harbour, so I had about half an hour to try to regain some energy for the evening.

The night progressed fairly well. When we arrived, there were photographers taking photos, then about an hour later the formal proceedings began. I was glad to find my seat after chatting with a few friends and staff members on the way in. Everyone seemed so happy to be finished with their exams. The stress was almost a distant memory.

Thankfully, I did not need to do much once I sat down, but there was a moment where each student was called up individually to receive a graduation certificate and shake the principal's hand. Our principal had a very gentle hand shake which was often the topic of conversation after anyone received an award at assembly, so everyone was going to get to experience it tonight. It is strange what things spark conversation amongst students ... even all these years later it stands out as a clear memory.

After the dinner the music was turned up and students were encouraged to dance. That was my queue to get going. I am not really a dancer and since getting sick I had become extra sensitive to noise, so once it became too hard to talk because the music was so loud, there was not a lot of point staying. I was quite exhausted by this point as well, so we made our way back to the car and I drifted off into my thoughts reflecting on the evening and the year that had been.

Another big end of school event was the Presentation Night. How different things were from just one year earlier! Being an annual event for K-12 it was not something specific to being in Year 12, but as a Year 12 student it was likely the last Presentation Night I would be involved in. I would get to be a spectator in future years as my sister continued at the school but this was my last chance to really be part of it. I was quite disappointed that this sickness would prevent me from enjoying it to the full. Nevertheless, I was determined to get there and hoped to participate in the Stage Band at least.

Award recipients are told they will be receiving an award a few days before the actual event and when I learnt that I would be receiving several awards I felt that strange mix of emotions resurface again ... mostly I felt that I did not deserve them ... how can I accept 'First place in ... anything' this year? Yet, I was thankful that I would still receive some awards because it had kind of become a bit of a tradition ... each year I seemed to do well academically and everyone came to expect it. Still, I knew that my good friend Linda had worked so hard and we were always so close in our marks – I hoped she would receive due recognition and we could be equal first place of subjects. As it turned out, my ranks from way back in June were preserved so I was awarded First place in Chemistry, Maths Extension 2 and Music 1. I was also awarded equal Dux – only not with Linda … she received 'Second place in Year 12'. Michelle, another one of my good friends, was equal Dux with me, so we were happy for her, but I still thought Linda should have got it.

When the actual night arrived, Tuesday December 11th, it was quite a different experience to what may have been. Instead of being in all the rehearsals leading up to the night and the whole day rehearsal on the day, I simply came when it was nearly time to begin. Mr Newton kindly allowed me to play for Stage Band. It was draining but I had enough adrenaline to get through the performances. Jess, one of my other friends who sings exceptionally well in the Stage Band and was also in Year 12, had a heavy cold and was barely able to talk let alone sing. She was pretty upset with how little voice she could get out for leading the opening song and she was not able to do much the rest of the night with her Stage Band song being scrapped for another one. Although completely different circumstances now someone else had a small taste of being in my shoes and I was able to try to encourage her in the moment.

The theme of the night was Amazing Grace. Despite all the challenges, it really was amazing to be there in the midst of it all and I knew that God's grace was carrying me through these difficult days. I was thankful to be part of it for one last time – thankfully the enemy could not rob me of that privilege. As the night drew to a close the Stage Band was back on stage for the big combined item "Light Surrounding You". After the farewell from the MCs, we launched into two more songs with Matt Corby (Year 11 student at our school who had come runner up in a very popular TV singing talent show that year) singing lead. That was a lot of fun and for a moment or two I was able to just enjoy playing trumpet with the group. Thank You for these blessings, Lord!

The final step to formally finishing Year 12 was to receive the HSC results and, even more significantly, to receive the all-important UAI.

Wednesday 19th December was the day for the release of the results. There was much anticipation because we would only find out the outcome of all our appeals for 'Illness/Misadventure' when the results were released! We had left that in God's hands. Surely, they would be accepted, right?

With a great sigh of relief, the results came through. They were fantastic! I again felt that my results were really Linda's (and Jess's for Music). Actually, they really *were* their results because the marks are based on the HSC exams which I didn't get to do. They did so well. My UAI was sky high too but only due to my peers putting in the hard yards when I could not continue.

It was a bit of a surreal moment. I had finally been awarded an HSC. One big chapter of my life was over. The next was about to begin ... yet I was still struggling to do little more than be awake.

When would the healing breakthrough come?
What was I to do?

Chapter 12:
Summer sorrows

The week before the HSC results came out, I received news about my audition to UNSW for the Bachelor of Music Bachelor of Education program. The email read: *"Unfortunately, you were unsuccessful in your recent audition with the School of Music and Music Education at the University of New South Wales for the BMus or BMusBEd or BMusBA course. The School of English, Media and Performing Arts: Music and Music Education offers music as a major strand within a Bachelor degree with two entry points that may offer you another means of studying music at university… The course Fundamentals of Music offers students a foundation in musicology and musicianship… you may also wish to audition again next year…"*

What???

It was like a punch to the stomach. I couldn't believe it. How can that be? I did not understand and couldn't make any sense of it. Surely with all my years of piano exams and musicianship exams I had a good enough foundation in musicology and musicianship.

I was gutted.

After all that effort and believing it was the right path to take … I didn't know what to do.

Mum was determined … it HAS to be a mistake! She set forth writing up a list of all my strengths and all our questions to ask why I was rejected and what exactly are the options for me to do now. She even thought to ask if I could be put on a waiting list if someone else pulled out.

I waited in anticipation as Mum phoned to find out ... yet another strange mix of emotions... disappointment, confusion, stress, anger, and yet still a tiny bit of hope that maybe Mum was right and it was a mistake ...

Well ... as it turned out, actually I was successful! The unsuccessful email WAS a mistake!

What a relief!!

Wow.

As the warm weather settled in for the summer, the length I had been sick ticked over the six-month mark and so the name for my mystery illness upgraded from post-viral fatigue to chronic fatigue syndrome. It was not an achievement I desired to be endowed with, but at least it was a more well-known and recognised issue than post-viral fatigue. That is, at least more people have heard of it. The condition itself had a lot of doubters – is it really something that engulfs people in an overwhelming fatigue ... or are these people just making it up? On the days I had a little more energy I had to battle with these thoughts myself even though I knew for sure that it was very real! How real?

Nowra ... our annual holiday. Every year since I was born our family had spent time in summer down the South coast of NSW at a place with a river... not just any river... the Shoalhaven River (or as I affectionally call it 'The Nowra River'). It was (and is) THE river for water skiers. Just ask our friends who make the 14-hour drive (almost) every year to holiday with us on the Shoalhaven River ... and ask them how many bridges over rivers they cross on their way down. Yep, Nowra is special.

Our time in Nowra typically consisted of boating, water skiing, teaching friends who visit how to water ski, tubing and wakeboarding (only if the water was no good for skiing!), early morning skis to get the best water (especially for those wanting to barefoot), deliberating what's for dinner with the other three or four families staying with us, boardgames, backyard (caravan park) cricket, watching the cricket, listening to the cricket up river on the boat radio and a bit of PS2. Oh, and the Mums made regular trips to the grocery stores to stock up our small fridges with an ample supply of food.

I had a lot of good memories from Nowra. When I was a young child Dad taught me to water ski and I loved it. Pre chronic fatigue days I would have been on the go the whole time we were out on the water – either behind the boat or in the water teaching someone to ski or in the boat observing (and taking photos) or driving (once I got my boat licence).

Nowra 2008 was markedly different. I spent a lot of time resting. I would lean on my pillow as we travelled up river to the beach. Then Dad would set up a camp stretcher for me to lie down to rest on the beach. Sometimes I would venture into the water and float on one of those body-length floatation devices, and other times if the boat was anchored, I would lie in the boat with the seats stretched out … just resting. It was tough watching everyone else have so much fun.

Dad knew I was sad to miss out and so he suggested I try to have just one little ski. How I longed to! But could I do it? Am I allowed to do it? Can someone with chronic fatigue do such things? Will it make me go backwards? Do I even have enough strength to hold onto the rope behind the boat? …

Dad reasoned that I was already tired so what did I have to lose … and besides that it is a long time before uni starts so I have plenty of time to recover any lost ground.

Well … only one way to find out …

Let's do it!

Honestly, I can't remember exactly how that ski went, but we do have a photo of it and I look exhausted! Usually, I look so happy and relaxed on the ski. I know that I was glad to have done it though and we all decided one was enough. Don't push it too much! Chronic fatigue indeed is a very real condition.

Despite a challenging summer, I did see improvement … Mum recorded in her journal *"God be praised. Dana definitely getting more energy, Rachel so thoughtful, caring, loving – Bible verses on healing decorating Dana's door with blue flowers. D awarded Academic Scholarship UNSW… Wore uniform last Sunday (church). Driven car 4 - 5x. Practising piano. Many signs of more strength and healing. Praise God."*

Chapter 13: A university student nonetheless

SEADU... Student Equity And Disability Unit. That was our destination for the day. It was Tuesday February 5th and our appointment was 9:30am at UNSW with Rita. This was just after the peak hour traffic, though still in the midst of the school drop off times. I am glad Mum was driving.

This was my first trip to the university. The campus was huge! So much bigger than my high school. Needless to say, we spent much time examining the campus map and planning the best place to park so that I would have the least distance to walk to the SEADU unit in the John Goodsell Building.

I was not too sure about signing up for disability provisions. I had started to improve a little since the end of 2007 and I did not want to take up services that other people may have needed more than me. Yet, I also knew that it would be better to set it all up for use while I continued to regain strength rather than starting with nothing and struggling because it was all too much. It was a very strange feeling to be coming into a place for the first time – no one knew who I was – and the first thing they learn about me was that I had chronic fatigue and needed SEADU help.

We made it through the traffic, found a carpark and found the building! First challenge completed. As it was only Summer Semester the campus was largely empty, but there was still an older lady sitting in a wheel-chair out the front of the building … smoking …

Ughh!!

I HATE the smell of cigarette smoke.

Even from a very young age I had always obviously hated the smell and tried so hard to avoid it at all costs. You would be hard pressed to find anything I disliked more. Mum and Dad were a little embarrassed at times with how strongly I would react, but there is just this righteous repulsiveness that comes over me every time – it would be dishonest and near impossible for me to react in any other way. I was a very good early detection system for them – they came to realise there was a smoker somewhere in the vicinity (often even a long way off) whenever I started to cough and pick up the pace to get past them fast into some fresher air again. I had this inbuilt warning system telling me that it was toxic. Please, if you do smoke – seek help to Quit – it will help your health immensely and will improve the health of those around you as well (not to mention it will also save you a lot of money).

The building was easily decades old … an old brown brick building with entrances on multiple levels, due to the university being built on a hill. To find Rita took a little longer than we would have liked, but eventually we found the section of the building where she was. Second challenge completed.

Mum did most of the talking and asking questions. She is very good at asking all the questions to get all the details. Rita discussed what provisions I could access and I had to sign a paper giving permission for my information to be shared across various sectors of the university. More people knowing my condition … I don't know about this … I suppose it would be helpful to not have to explain it to everyone. Third challenge completed. Let's go home for a rest!

The following week my GP supplied a letter of support explaining my condition and requesting provisions that Rita had recommended. His support had been so helpful during my whole time of sickness. He didn't know how to fix the problem, but he was supportive in providing all the documentation we needed and as a Christian he could pray as well. One line in his last paragraph was hard to swallow though, *"it would be reasonable to assume that she will continue to be significantly disabled for the whole of this academic year."* Please let that not be true, Lord.

Once Rita had received the GP letter, she compiled a letter for those that needed to know so that my special provisions would be put in place. I was provided note-takers for lectures, use of a locker, resting room access, an academic liaison, and recommendations for exam support.

After another visit to Rita on the 19th of February it seemed to be all sorted out. I also was able to meet the Head of the degree I was enrolled in that morning. He would be teaching Music Reinvented (one of the subjects for Semester 1) as well so I now had met one of my lecturers.

The next big thing was O-Week… That is 'Orientation Week', also known as 'Week Zero'. I had missed the Faculty of Arts and Social Sciences Advising Day on the 12th of February as I did not want to overdo it before uni even started! Monday and Thursday were the days I needed to be at O-Week. How different to school which is Monday to Friday week in and week out!

O-Week was the week for signing up to anything and everything. All the student-led clubs and groups were out in force with their marquees lining the main walkway at the bottom of the university ... just before the dreaded 200 steps which lead to the upper level of the university.

Yes, you read that correctly. 200 steps.

I remember one night explaining it to my sister at the dinner table....

"So, Matthews is the top of the juice?" asked Rachel.

Hmmm. What else is taller, I thought as I shook my head and peered around the table. Aha! The water bottle.

"No, the end of the 200 stairs is the top of the juice ... The table cloth is the bus stop, the height of the cup is lower campus, the lids of the salt and pepper shakers are Central Lecture Block, the top of the juice is the Library, which is in upper campus and is pretty much the top of the 200 stairs. The lid on top of the water bottle is the lecture halls in Matthews," I answered.

My sister was taking it all in ...

"It's a lot bigger than high-school!" I added to re-emphasise the point.

Thankfully, there were routes which helped to avoid the majority of these steps if you were unfortunate enough to have a class at either end of the uni back-to-back ... or in my case I would need the shortcuts every time so I didn't get stuck somewhere on the steps and just need to lie down. I got quite good at the shortcut over my time at the university and taught quite a few fellow students the secret to avoiding the giant staircase.

Option A: Walk into the Electrical Engineering Building, take the lift to Level 2, take the ramp to the John Goodsell Building (I think you needed an access pass to get in that entrance), take the lift to Level 1 and you had made it to the top of the stairs with 0 stairs climbed.

Option B: Take the 200 stairs.

Option C: Walk up the side of the 200 stairs on the steep, wide footpath ramp.

Obviously, I had to do Option A every time, until I regained enough strength to hand back the access pass and I then did a modified route which had about 30 steps to do rather than the 200. Option D was to be dropped off at the top of the campus and walk down to the buildings, but this was not possible if there was a class in lower campus first.

Anyway, back to O-Week. I enjoyed perusing the many marquees but knew that at this stage they were all out of the question for me. The waterskiing one was tempting. Maybe one day ... I hoped. There was also CBS ... Campus Bible Study. I would like to try that someday too if I get enough energy. At that stage my energy levels would only allow me to come to uni for my timetabled classes and go straight home.

Due to my lingering lack of energy Dad worked so hard at scheduling his out of office jobs in line with my university schedule so that he could drive me to and from uni on the days Mum was at work. If Mum was not working, she would drive me to and from uni. The support of my parents was amazing.

I was also super excited to find out that not one, not two, but three of my close high school friends were attending UNSW! Wow! So cool. Michelle, Lucy and Linda. Yes, Linda, the one who had been in almost all my classes and had taken notes for me and kept me in the loop with everything school related throughout my sickness. She was now enrolled in a Chemical Engineering degree. So, while we did not have any university classes together, it was great to be able to catch up for lunch if we had a break at the same time. We would also try and coordinate with Lucy and Michelle. So lovely to have some familiar faces around the (huge) new place.

As I sat through one of the Music introductory classes I learnt of the requirement for ALL students to be involved in at least one large music ensemble and one small ensemble. That was going to be a BIG stretch ... maybe impossible at this stage. The large music ensembles were orchestra, wind band or choir. It would have been great fun to be in wind band, but all three large ensembles had long late afternoon or night-time rehearsals. There was no way I could be out for long days or out late at night and then up early in the morning for university the next day. I could only cope with a few hours at a time and going home and coming back again was also fairly difficult because I was relying on Mum and Dad for all my transport still as I was not up to driving that far, especially at the end of the classes for the day. The small ensembles were mostly held over lunchbreaks so I could see potential for being able to participate in them.

Now I was thankful for the SEADU process I had gone through and I petitioned to have a special provision of joining two small ensembles instead of a large one and a small one. Thankfully, my petition was granted and I joined Handbells and Jazz Fundamentals. Handbells was great. It was something I had never seen let alone tried before. Each bell represented a different pitch (like a different key on the piano). Each person was given about four bells to cover. You had to read the music score and ring one of your four or so bells at the appropriate moment so that it sounded like a song and not like a dog's breakfast! It required concentration and skill, and it was a lot of fun learning new songs as we all tried hard not to mess up. I was even able to get the group to play one of my high school music compositions as it was something achievable for the group to learn. However, as it had an Alberti bass if you had one of the repeating notes you got a tired arm rather quickly! (Alberti bass is where the notes keep repeating in a consistent pattern over and over and over again).

To my surprise and delight one of the other people in the handbells group was Rach, one of my Nana's other pupils. Nana conducted private music tuition for piano, singing and music theory/musicianship. Rach was a singer further along in her degree. Again, it was so nice to see a familiar face in those early days at uni.

Jazz Fundamentals was also quite fun … until it was your turn to do an improvised solo! I did want to get better at it, but also found it a bit daunting playing an improvisation in front of everyone … at least it couldn't really be wrong as it was made up on the spot! Some 'solos' definitely sounded a lot better than others though!!

Anyone could join the music ensembles and you could play whichever instrument you wanted to, so although Michelle was not studying music at university she came along for the group and it was great to spend time together again. Michelle would often play keyboard and I would play trumpet.

In a future semester at uni, I joined Gypsy Jazz because the Jazz Fundamentals did not line up with the rest of my timetable. Gypsy Jazz was much harder than Jazz Fundamentals! Most of the group played a guitar and transposing the 'licks' (musical phrases) involved moving up or down a fret. I was on the trumpet however, and this involved intense mental gymnastics playing in keys with lots of sharps and then transposing, sometimes on the spot! Very challenging!!

Chapter 14:
Challenges and blessings

With the special provision for the ensembles in place and my parents driving me I sailed through the first semester fairly well. The biggest challenge was Professional Experience. I needed to attend a primary school for five days a week for three weeks, observing, assisting and then teaching as per the requirements outlined for us. It was going to be a big test of my endurance.

The university asked us to choose a school and liaise with them in order to organise the placement. I chose to return to my old primary school. It was very close to home so that would help reduce the energy loss from travel, and it was a school I was familiar with so I would need less energy compared to being in a completely new setting.

Wow. Going back to primary school! How crazy. I never thought I would be back to teach at my primary school. We were asked to do a primary school first because music was a K-12 subject, though our degree was primarily training us for secondary teaching.

"4J" was the name of the class I was given. They were a beautiful class and at such a nice age. They were far easier to teach than the young ones in infants as they were able to learn many things yet they did not have the arrogant attitude that some of the Year 6 students displayed. That being said, it was still a big learning curve and definitely challenging at times to get the class to listen and participate sensibly. Overall though, the class seemed to enjoy the experience as music is not often a big focus for primary schools (especially within the classroom) so it was something special for them. From recorders to brass instruments, from Baroque to Classical, from musicals to jazz, we explored a wide range of instruments, songs, styles and genres!

During the prac I was able to observe concert band rehearsals and they even happened to have a special 'Performing Arts Assembly' at that time. Sitting through the usual weekly assembly brought back many memories – the structure was almost identical to how it had been all those years ago... "Welcome to this week's assembly..." one of the student leaders began... it was so familiar I almost forgot I was not still a student!

At one of these regular weekly assemblies, two of the students from 4J performed. They did a great job. I did make a note in my prac diary though that I should *"Perhaps mention to performers that it's good to adjust/alter the music a little so audience doesn't have to count rests. The audience may think you are lost or that you are finished if there are big gaps."* Haha, yes, I never thought that would need explaining, but now I know it does.

At the end of the three weeks, I gave the students a note...

"Thank you for having me in your classroom over the last 3 weeks. I enjoyed teaching you music and hope you enjoyed learning from me. Congratulations to all who performed in our '4J's Got Talent – Celebration of Music'. Performing in front of your peers is a difficult task, so well done. Your composing skills impressed me and our mini-musical 'Little Red Riding Hood' was fantastic! I encourage you to keep on learning your music."

The class presented me with a hand-made 'Thank You' card which had a photo of the class and myself on the front, and on the inside was a message from the classroom teacher and the students had also signed it. Such a lovely memento. I finished off the prac with "Friday afternoon sport" and then headed home ready for a holiday period I definitely needed … a time to rest, recuperate and hopefully be ready for Semester 2.

Towards the end of Semester my wrists and forearms had really started to get sore.

"My wrists just hurt so much," I complained to Mum.

"Look, I can only bend them this far", I despaired as I struggled to get them past the horizontal …

This was not good … especially for my Major, Piano. Mum booked me in to get checked out during the holidays. Yay … just what I needed … more medical appointments. I was able to hit a trifecta the week before uni returned … GP, ultrasound and hand therapist.

"So, I've got to wear these for two weeks?" I asked Lisa, the hand therapist.

"Yes, wear the wrist braces as much as possible, 24/7 for two weeks. Do not use your fingers or your wrists. Keep as still as possible," she replied. "After that we will review and hopefully reduce the amount of time you need to keep them on per day."

The braces were wetsuit material with Velcro to hold them in place as they wrapped around your hand and half-way up your lower arm. They wrapped around between the thumb and index finger. There was a firm metal rod holding the wrist in a slightly upward position. It was intended to give the tendons time to relax and de-stress. They had become so tense from overuse that they simply would not stretch, so I could not bend my wrist downwards at all.

Yes, I had to wear them on both arms … I had the problem in both wrists. How???

Piano.

Apparently, the increase in practicing piano as part of my university degree had brought the onset of tendonitis in both wrists. The ultrasound report called it 'tenosynovitis'. Was this related to chronic fatigue? I have no idea. Maybe because I had stopped practicing for several months, I may have lost the stamina I had built up over the years and perhaps the weakening of my muscles overall had contributed. Whatever the case, it was NOT helpful.

I ended up requesting to change my major instrument from piano to trumpet … to be honest, this was a bit of a leap of faith. I had never done any trumpet exams and never practiced any scales or other technical work. I had never had any formal trumpet lessons. I had just picked it up in primary school for concert band so I could also play it at church and then I played it at high school over the years.

How hard can it be?

Well, first I had to find a trumpet teacher as the university required us to be getting weekly private tuition for our major instrument. Mr Newton to the rescue! Ironically, he had also studied the same degree at the same university with the same major (trumpet) so he was very familiar with all the processes required. He found some suitable pieces and we got to work.

The problem was that trumpet took a much greater physical toll on the body in terms of energy output. My endurance for the lessons and practicing at home needed much improvement. Still, at least I could continue my studies. There was no way the hand therapist was going to let me practice piano any time soon!

Aside from the wrist braces I also had to go to regular physio appointments to massage out the knots. The hand therapist was the physio. She had treated a range of people over the years and even the big tough footy players would often be in tears with her massage treatment ... when the knots were pushed up through the arm towards the tip of the elbow the pain skyrocketed! It was like a Chinese burn with a very firm pinch at the same time. Owww! It was awful!

Fast forward to mid-2009 and it was time for our second year prac. The butterflies in my stomach started to flutter as the time drew nearer. We all knew it was coming. I, and several other students in my degree, approached prac a bit like how I approached swimming lessons. Back in the day when I went for weekly swimming lessons at the local pool, I would dread the thought of going there ... it seemed like so much effort to pack the swimming bag, travel there, get changed, get in the water, do all the training, get dry and changed again, then travel home. Think of all the other productive and fun things I could have done in that time and with less effort! Yet, I did actually enjoy it once I was in the water, and being able to confidently swim is definitely a great skill to have. Prac was like that. I didn't like the thought of it and all the effort it would involve, but I did *mostly* enjoy the experience once I was there.

I chose to do prac at my old high school. Yes, the school where my chronic fatigue began. Well, technically it was post-viral fatigue still when I graduated, but we all know that was just the name you used until the six-month mark.

I was both apprehensive and excited to return. I was thankful for the opportunity to 'finish' there in a better state. Though I was not 100 percent yet, my last memory of high school would no longer need to be 'never finishing year 12'. Rather, it could be 'second year prac'. God is so kind to orchestrate things like this for us. He is the God of Redemption.

Mr Newton was assigned as my supervising teacher. Most of my high school teachers were still there. It was such a blessing, such a special moment to enter the main staffroom that first morning and join in with staff prayer. We broke off into small groups and prayed with one another and for one another. There was no better way I could think of to start off prac.

The blessings kept coming. It was Mission Week during my prac. This was a once-a-year event in which the school had a big focus on evangelism to the students. There would be a theme, competitions with prizes, a devotional and inspirational booklet given to every student which was to be worked through during homegroup time, the special assemblies in which there would be special guests (speakers, musicians etc), and there would be an extended lunch with many fun activities for the students to participate in. What a privilege to be part of it all. I was asked to make a CD (yes, this was before digital music took over everything) for an 'air guitar' competition which would run during the special assembly. That was a fiddly project to do … getting the exact excerpts of each song down on separate tracks … I was pleased to be able to help though. At the staff meeting the Monday morning after Mission Week we learnt that 10 students desired to become a Christian (many from the Senior School), about 40 students had questions about Christianity and about 40 had struggles they wanted help with. What a great response! Praise God!

My sister was still at the school, so that was another fun aspect of this prac. Plus, I did know some of the students from being in the musical groups together during my time at the school. Attending Stage Band rehearsals brought back lots of memories. Also, during my prac I took part in a special evening concert with the Stage Band and a recently made famous singer/trumpeter, Carl Risely.

Teaching the classes was a learning curve again. High school students are quite different to the Year 4 class I had the year before in my first prac. It was a gentle introduction to the high school dynamics though because this was a familiar school for me and an Independent School which meant the students were generally fairly well behaved.

Towards the end of the prac my former maths teacher invited me to let them know if I wanted any casual work. This was a kind offer, but I knew that my health still needed some improvement, so rather than trying to over extend myself I knew I needed to focus on completing uni before looking at work.

Chapter 15:
A whiff of normality

In July 2009 we headed North. It was a rather common occurrence for our family to head North in the Winter holidays to visit our relatives in Queensland. These were always exciting times as often we would visit a theme park or two and I even looked forward to and enjoyed the all-day trips in the car to get there and get home.

Dad loved driving so the all-day trip in the car was quite enjoyable for him as well. He did not like stopping though, so it was often two stops. One for a late (second) breakfast. (The first breakfast was around 4am before we got in the car to begin the big drive.) The second stop was for lunch, usually around Coffs Harbour, but as the road incorporated more bypasses this eventually became a late lunch at the Gold Coast!

Mum mostly slept and my sister would get through the day with a mixture of sleep, listening to the amazing 'Odyssey' tapes (Bible stories on cassette tapes – yes there were still cassette tapes around then!), doing something creative with me like creating a puppet show for our cousins, or being the cymbal as I played the 'air drums' along to the music we were listening to in the car ... usually brass band, songster (church choir) songs or singing company (kids church choir) songs. It was lots of fun. She was very accommodating letting me use her shoulder as the cymbal. Don't worry, I was very gentle!

The 2009 trip didn't disappoint. We had gone to Qld in 2008 as well, but I was still being quite cautious and struggling with my energy levels back then. One of the highlights for 2009 was MovieWorld. It had been some time since we had been to a theme park and my favourite was Dreamworld, then SeaWorld, then MovieWorld. I think we may have only done Wet 'n' Wild twice over the years. So, MovieWorld didn't get much of a look in, but we decided because we had not been there for so long and there was a new "Superman Escape" rollercoaster to try that we should make MovieWorld and SeaWorld the theme parks for this year. Dreamworld missed out.

First up was MovieWorld. We got through the park gates and picked up the map ready to plan our day. Soon enough we learnt that the "Lethal Weapon" ride was closed for renovations. That was a bit of a let down because that was Dad's favourite ride at the park … One day I hoped to be brave enough to go on it with him, but alas, this was not the year for it. I'm fairly comfortable to go on most rides, but this one was just a bit more extreme … It was a roller-coaster with no carriage – that is, you just were strapped into a seat with your legs dangling. The track was above your head … *"Lethal Weapon offers the most awesome thrill ride experience featuring over 765m of non-stop drops, dives, bends, rollovers, sidewinders, double spins, loops and plungers … you'll see your feet against the sky, travel at 85km/h and feel 4Gs of gravity!"* boasted the MovieWorld brochure … ok, so maybe it was a good thing it was closed. Face that fear another day!

But … the new Superman Escape rollercoaster was open! The MovieWorld brochure set the scene for us … *"Welcome to the world's most AWESOME rollercoaster experience –*

SUPERMAN ESCAPE. Escape a terrifying earthquake in the METROPOLIS subway as the world's coolest Super Hero propels you vertically upwards at 100km/h – in 2 seconds! Then experience an exhilarating and hair raising rollercoaster ride experience like no other".

Rach and Mum were not such thrill seekers and easily made the choice to pass on that one. Dad and I though, we were very keen! We headed over to the ride and ...

What a big queue!! Dad hates queues. I looked up at him and asked hesitatingly ... "Should we wait?"

He thought about it ... we looked at the rollercoaster ... we deliberated ...

We waited ... for over an hour!

But it was worth it!

That acceleration was something else!! It would have been great to go on it again, but we were not standing in the queue for another hour! Time to go find Mum and Rach and do some rides together.

We made our way to the Wild West Falls Adventure Ride. This was like a log flume where you sit in a little boat that is taken along a little creek and eventually you come to a giant drop in which some or all of the riders get wet ... or very wet! Over the years we came to expect Mum to get the wettest on these rides. Somehow, she always managed to get the seat that was the perfect position to receive the biggest deluge of water.

Well, we all got rather wet, Mum included. It was a fun ride.

Scooby Doo Spooky Coaster was bizarre. It was also quite a long wait, but at least we were together. It was another rollercoaster, but with little carriages and a narrow windy track inside a building. It was quite dark inside and the ride jolted us around a lot. We were going not too bad until the ride halted and then suddenly went backwards! That took us all by surprise! Rachel and Mum particularly did not like that. We all thought it should have had a higher thrill rating than the park let on. Definitely a memorable one, but not really that enjoyable.

We enjoyed the Hollywood Stunt Driver show as a family, Dad and I had a go at the Batwing Spaceshot and the Shrek 4D adventure was a nice way for the four of us to end the day as we were able to sit down and rest a bit as we watched the show. The special effects were quite clever making you feel like you were almost in the movie. It had been good to be able to enjoy the day together as a family and the chronic fatigue barely rated a mention.

We also went jet-skiing while we were up there. This was so much fun. Although I had to wear my wrist braces still, and despite the speed limiter as they were hire jet skis, it was great to get out on the water and experience the twists and turns and feel the spray – in winter! So nice to get some sunshine and warmth up in QLD.

We found a Mini Golf which was fun for the whole family, and SeaWorld was great to be at again after several years. There was a new ride called Jet Rescue. It rivalled the Superman Escape for acceleration! Maybe not quite as fast, but it really was a unique experience as the ride seat was to sit on a jet ski which then went around the rollercoaster track. That was great fun! We also went on an old favourite The Bermuda Triangle ride, got drenched on the simple but effective old Viking's Revenge Log Flume and thoroughly enjoyed watching the very talented skiers in the Waterskiing show. It was almost like old times. I began to realise I was feeling good ... I began to believe that maybe I had turned the corner ...

Was I ok now?

Was the chronic fatigue almost gone?

Chapter 16:
The foolish wisdom teeth

on't make me laugh!" …

"Please!"

It was mid-July 2009. My sister had just returned home from a camp. I was lying on the couch recovering from surgery. Wisdom teeth removal to be precise.

Mum gave Rachel 'the stare' indicating she better not make me laugh.

Rachel glanced over at me and tried really hard to hold it in, but the smile just spread across her face from ear to ear and she burst out laughing …

And, of course, laughter is contagious and so there was no hope for me to stop the inevitable …

"Ouch!" …

"Rachel!" I exclaimed as I tried to ease the pain after the laughing episode.

"I'm sorry … you just look so funny like that … your cheeks!" … she muffled through more laughter that she tried to suppress.

"It's not funny!" I tried to convince her, and myself …

It had been a few days now and the swelling just would not go down. My cheeks were so swollen that it looked like I had a tennis ball stuffed into each side of my mouth! It was a ridiculous sight! I couldn't really blame her for laughing. But the tension in my cheeks was right on the limit and any further stretch, such as the motion of smiling or laughing, caused an onslaught of pain.

The actual surgery had taken place on 13th July and we were only proceeding with it because we were advised that it was necessary. Yes, apparently leaving them there would potentially cause problems and it was necessary that not one or two but all four wisdom teeth be removed. So, I had to go to a hospital and I had to go under for it. That was the first time I had received a general anaesthetic. I was not looking forward to it – as you know, I hate needles! And I was a little apprehensive with the unknown, but armed with prayer and reassurance from family it all proceeded rather well on the day. The hardest part was trying to take a drink of water before I could be discharged … apparently the anaesthetic had not worn off enough at the first attempt and the water dribbled out of my mouth everywhere. What a mess! It was not too long though before I was successful and could go home.

The problems started to be apparent in the following days … the swelling in my face was so persistent … it just would not budge. I was swollen for weeks on end! It also took nearly two weeks for my back teeth to be able to close again so I was on a soft food diet for quite some time. The toll on my body was significant and I was very weak for several days after the operation. The chronic fatigue must have been holding on still. Although I was not back to square one the recovery took a long time and even when I was 'recovered' it seemed like I had taken a backward step from how good I was feeling during our Queensland trip.

One thing was certain, I was definitely not in a hurry to have any more visits to the hospital!

By September I had enough energy to take part in the church brass band trip to Tuggeranong to do concerts at a church, the Floriade flower festival and Bunnings! How random! Each venue was quite different to the others but it was a lot of fun. It was also great to have the opportunity to encourage each other in our faith as we spent time with one another over the weekend. Reflecting on it all I was grieved that so many people had left the church … why would anyone want to leave? Did they not know what God offers us? As I read the Scriptures that night God highlighted a verse that really resonated with me, especially with how I had been reflecting on the weekend … *"But my life is worth nothing to me unless I use it for finishing the work assigned me by the Lord Jesus – the work of telling others the Good News about the wonderful grace of God." (Acts 20:24, NLT).* What a testimony, what a verse to live by!

Chapter 17:
Summer sorrows return

At the end of November, I had a relapse of chronic fatigue. Was it the wisdom teeth removal? I think it is highly likely that was a contributor ... but whatever the case this *was* like going back to square one.

All the progress I had made ... gone.

The overwhelming tiredness settled in for a long, very tired summer. Almost two and a half years since the start of this illness and it was like it was starting all over again.

No!

I will not be like this the rest of my life.

It was a real battle to not get totally deflated, but I had this determination, like I had had since the start of the illness, that I would be healed of it someday. I was definitely disappointed, upset, confused and angry that I was back in such a weak, exhausted state, but I was fighting for healing.

This relapse solidified two things for me. Number one – it really was 'that bad'. During the two and a half years I had had good days and bad days and as I improved it was hard to imagine how bad the bad days really were. The psychological battle would come back – was it really bad enough to keep me out of school that long? Was it really bad enough to stop me doing so many things? This relapse gave a resounding YES! Now I had no doubt that it was that bad.

Number two – I needed to get better.

By the time Nowra arrived in January I was still rather exhausted, but I managed to have a few skis. Not the usual quota, but more than one. I waited for the good water and made the most of the few skis I was able to have ... complete with wrist braces as I was still needing support there as well. I also managed to drive the boat a few times, so it was better than the 2008 edition of Nowra.

These excerpts from my journal show the struggle I was in...

2nd January 2010

"Lord, You know what I'm going through. You've heard my thoughts and prayers. Help me to keep enduring – being patient and holding on to the hope You've given me! In Jesus' name, Amen"

16th January 2010

"Thank You Father God for Your Word and Your promises. I pray for strength for this day – may I live how You want and to praise and glorify You always..."

30th January 2010

"Help me to always come to You for help"

9th February 2010

"Please give me strength for this day..."

20th February 2010

"I ask for strength for the BBQ ... tonight and strength for church tomorrow. In Jesus' name"

23rd February 2010

"Thank You for helping me through so many hard situations since November when I've felt a real lack of energy

on most days. I want to live Your way – to do Your will and trust You despite my circumstances – You can do all things – I ask for strength and healing. In Jesus' name, Amen."

The following weekend was Youth Councils. This is a special event within the Salvation Army where the Youth Groups from churches across the city (or state) join together to worship Jesus, have fun, get to know more people and hear guest speakers share the Word of God. At 20, I was getting to the older end of the 'Youth' but still young enough to be involved. I made it for the Sunday morning session. The guest speaker this year was from America. It was the testimony from local Aussie, Nathan Hodges, though that stood out to me. He shared that God can give us specific answers in miraculous ways ... but we need to actually ask Him the questions first! *"you do not have because you do not ask. You ask and do not receive, because you ask amiss, that you may spend it on your pleasures."* (James 4:2b-3)

Nathan had asked God a specific question and out of the blue a Christian leader who knew nothing of his journey came up to him and said "God said to say, 'Yes'." I reflected in my journal and decided to write out my pressing questions to the Lord.

28th February 2010

"That's so amazing and I believe You can answer my questions too! Help me to listen to Your answers. You already know my questions, but You want me to ask You :) So here are the things I'm not sure about:

- *Should I persist with the naturopath, Claudette? Do we trust her unlabelled bottle?*
- *Should I do uni fully this year? Or look at maybe not doing one or two subjects to ease the physical workload?*

-   *What should I do about worship team and band at church? I'd love to be in both, especially band, but I want to do Your will and be able to grow by being fed – not getting all worn out on these extra things. I want to worship You and serve You how You want.*

Father – they are the main questions – You know what's best so help me to obey You. I ask You in Jesus' name for healing to my body as well and for answers to those questions. Help me to listen and to grow, to read Your Word and pray and be a real witness for You. I want to reach others for Your kingdom! In Jesus' name, Amen."

Chapter 18:
He will direct your paths

It did not take long for God to move after writing out those questions. The most significant moment of my journey was about to unfold.

March 2010. An epoch in time that I will forever be thankful for.

"Dana, Aunty Jody found a book from Koorong that she wants to send you. I know you don't like to read all that much but she said she believes it's really important."

I was intrigued. Yes, I'm not much of a reader. I really struggled to read those compulsory novels for English in high school and I detested reading through all the irrelevant research we had to do at uni, but I did enjoy reading the Bible, testimonies and devotionals.

I looked over at Mum lost in my thoughts still ... Another thing to try ... am I ready for this? If it's from Koorong (Christian bookstore) it might be worth a read ...

"Well, if she's already bought it for me, I guess I should try and read it."

A few days later the book arrived and I glanced at the title *Daniel's Diet Lifestyle*. There was a giant metallic spoon on the front cover with three brilliantly bright red raspberries on it. Behind the spoon was a yellow bowl filled with the rest of the raspberries. The majority of the book cover was a crisp, clean white. Along the bottom of the cover were four rectangular pictures – someone drinking a glass of juice, a lettuce leaf, a man running by the ocean, and a close up of blueberries.

It's about food.

Memories of the mean doctor who jabbed me in 'my arm not his' came flooding back. I have already tried changing my diet and it did nothing for me …

The subtitle of the book read "Restoring God's health plan". Maybe this time it will be different.

I opened the cover and Aunty Jody had left me a message… *"I was in Koorong the other day and felt the Holy Spirit ask me to buy you this book. I didn't look inside it until I was outside the shop, sitting down for morning tea. I saw that the first page explained how the author successfully treated chronic fatigue patients and I knew this book was for you!"*

Now that got my attention!

God told her to buy it, and the author had a track record of seeing chronic fatigue patients get healed. Wow! *"Trust in the Lord with all your heart, And lean not on your own understanding; In all your ways acknowledge Him, And He shall direct your paths." (Proverbs 3:5-6).*

I definitely wanted to read it now.

Chapter One began with the words that were like music to my ears… *"This 'mysterious' illness was causing much community concern for it was almost impossible to diagnose and was deemed incurable by most authorities. However, as it turned out, three diagnosed chronic fatigue sufferers came to consult with me in a two-week period and I soon discovered that with a determined lifestyle change, these 'so-called' incurable cases dramatically improved. The lifestyle changes included natural supplements and a specific cleansing and rebuilding diet…*

I was compelled to write a research paper that demonstrated the Chronic Fatigue Syndrome (CFS/ME) was a real and significant problem. I wished to inform people that there was help available to give them hope and a direction to follow ...

Then I discovered a diet that was 2500 years old.

After treating many people with ME (CFS) and various other illnesses I began to realise there was a missing link in the overall recovery of some patients ... the 'spiritual side' of the holistic approach to healing". (Bridgeman, 2005, p.11-12)

The author, Philip, then went on to describe how God sent him a Christian secretary which eventually resulted in him becoming a Christian too. His life dramatically changed and he... *"had discovered the missing link, the link to true holistic health and healing – Jesus Christ and the Cross."* (Bridgeman, 2005, p.12)

I was captivated and becoming excited at the possibilities ... thank You Lord, show me what I need to do here please.

Philip went on to explain the Biblical plan for diet and health in a way that made so much sense but just is not really talked about much ... or at least I had never heard it taught before. People love to eat whatever they like and so when you start to touch on what we eat as being a part of our Christian walk it is not received well ... 'everything in moderation' is the old adage that people just fall back on ... But is that what God's Word teaches?

No! God teaches that we need to look after our body as it is the temple of the Holy Spirit. He teaches that there are certain foods that are not good for us. He teaches that we will reap what we sow.

"So, If You Are Sick:
1.   Turn to Jesus – Matthew 8:16, 17. 1 Peter 2:24

2. *Pray and be prayed for by your church and friends. (James 5:14, 15, 16). Learn to find and declare (stand on) your own scriptures and believe in faith (not just repetitious quoting of scripture- but deep heart belief.) ...*

3. *Change your lifestyle and diet – work with Jesus in your healing, not against Him. Put your faith into action. To expect God to heal us when we deliberately ignore the principles (laws) He has laid down for our health is really being disobedient. It is not enough that God wills our health – we must will it also."* (Bridgeman, 2005, p.23-24)

Now there's an action plan! I had turned to Jesus, I had been praying for healing and was being prayed for. I had been standing on promises but maybe not whole-heartedly. Point three was where it suddenly started to make sense. *"Work with Jesus in your healing, not against Him."* (Bridgeman, 2005, p.23) When I had done the dietary changes with the mean doctor there were no explanations as to why and there was no focus on living in obedience to the Scriptures, nor any emphasis on the power of eating in a truly healthy way to help the body get what it needed to have the best opportunity for recovery.

I kept reading ... and reading ... I couldn't read it all in one sitting because there was a lot to digest and I was also still struggling with my energy levels. But within one to three weeks, I had completed reading the book and had begun to implement changes to my diet.

Romans 12:2 says *"And do not be conformed to this world, but be transformed by the renewing of your mind, that you may prove what is that good and acceptable and perfect will of God."* As I read the book my mind was being transformed. I was gaining a new understanding about the goodness contained in the foods God had provided for us to eat. In turn, I began to desire to try more fruit and vegetables, nuts and grains which previously I had written off as something I would never like or would not be bothered to try. I also began to put away the junk food that I would snack on. My desire for it greatly decreased it once I knew it was not helping my body be healthy. Before reading the book, I thought I ate reasonably healthy and didn't know there were any problems with it. The Bible warns us about this too... *"My people are destroyed for lack of knowledge"* (Hosea 4:6a) ... But if we *"shall know the truth, {then} the truth shall make you free."* (see John 8:32)

So, what is the truth? Our modern lifestyle and diet subject our bodies to multitudes of toxins daily. This leads to all manner of illness and physical problems. *"God's provision and counterbalance is in His food. In natural food, along with supplements, we can find everything we need to combat all the toxins and resultant ill health... Comprehend this fact and it should forever make you want to eat more of the natural foods ... eat foods with life in them."* (Bridgeman, 2005, p.38)

Just as Jesus' words are spirit and they are life (see John 6:63), the foods God has created for us to eat are life for our bodies. For example, there are antioxidants, vitamins and minerals, phyto-nutrients, biologically active substances, fibre, natural sugars, and enzymes found in food. These are all necessary for the body to function well. (Bridgeman, 2005)

A couple of foods on my 'I should try and eat them even though I didn't previously like them' list were beetroot and rockmelon. Beetroot has so many health benefits I simply could not ignore it, from detoxifying the blood to replenishing vitamins, minerals, enzymes and natural sugars, and it contains compounds to fight cancer and inhibit tumours! (Bridgeman, 2005, p.40) Rockmelon was listed as a food that reduces risk of cancer and heart disease, plus provides significant levels of Vitamin C, potassium and beta-carotenes. (Bridgeman, 2005, p.41) I also learnt that each colour of food represents a different combination of health benefits, so variety is important in our eating. (Bridgeman, 2005).

I began to discuss what I was learning from the book with Mum. She found it interesting too, but I don't think she was grasping it as well as me. I guess there was a lot more at stake for me so I was like a sponge ready to soak up all the knowledge I could!

One day soon after completing the book I worked up the courage to ask Mum the question I had been pondering in my mind for some time...

Chapter 19:
Dare to be a Daniel

"Can I do the Daniel's Diet detox please Mum?"

The Daniel's Diet detox was a big catalyst for the change which the *Daniel's Diet Lifestyle* book had provided many testimonies of. Changing my eating habits was a good start, but if I wanted a clean slate for my body to rebuild, a detox was the answer. Clean out the rubbish and rebuild with good, life-giving foods.

Mum took some time to think it through and surprised me with her response "Of course darling… and I will do it with you too."

I was amazed at Mum's willingness to jump in and do it with me.

We got to work planning out our 10-day Daniel detox. The detox is based on the story of Daniel in Scripture. Daniel 1 to be precise, although Daniel and his friends were not using it as a detox, they were using it to prove God and His ways are better than the pagan Babylonian gods and their system which Daniel and his friends, as captives, were under. *"But Daniel purposed in his heart that he would not defile himself with the portion of the king's delicacies, nor with the wine which he drank"* (Daniel 1:8a) Daniel asked his superior *"Please test your servants for ten days, and let them give us vegetables to eat and water to drink. Then let our appearance be examined before you, and the appearance of the young men who eat the portion of the king's delicacies; and as you see fit, so deal with your servants."* (Daniel 1:12-13) It required a resolute, strong uncompromising faith. If Daniel and his friends looked weaker than the other young men after 10 days of eating God's diet, they likely would have been killed. But they looked better than all the rest after the 10 days.

God blessed them for their uncompromising obedience and faith.

Although Daniel had a lot more on the line, this detox for me was also about obedience and faith ... obedience to act on what I was learning about the foods God has provided us with and having faith that God can heal me. As well as obedience and faith, the key to doing this Daniel diet detox well would be preparation. Whilst you could just eat fresh fruit, raw, steamed and roast vegetables, it would be a bit boring randomly picking whatever was available and eating just that for 10 days straight. It also would likely not get the variety necessary to get all the vitamins, minerals and enzymes our bodies need. Some (most) people also need something to help clean out their intestines to allow the body to detox.

The book came with instructions on what we could and could not include during the 10 days. The 'No' foods were dairy, grains (except brown rice and millet), caffeine, yeast, sugar, fried foods, artificial chemicals, shop bought sauces/gravies/spreads, eggs, meat, white rice, table salt, alcohol. That rules out a lot of what people eat these days! The 'Yes' foods were vegetables, vegetable juices, nuts and seeds, fruit, brown (or basmati) rice, millet, dandelion coffee, herbal teas, water, and natural sweeteners (a little) if you are really struggling to get off the sugar. (Bridgeman, 2005, p.55-70)

Hmmm.

I don't know if I had ever had a meal with only the yes foods in it! Still, I was feeling fairly positive about it all.

Thankfully the book also included a sample detox plan and a bunch of recipes to get us started. Mum and I perused the recipes and came up with our own Daniel's Diet 10-day detox schedule.

Philip encouraged those bold enough to take on the challenge… *"Enjoy the experience, experiment with different foods, see and feel the benefits of de-toxing and feeling clean and healthy."* (Bridgeman, 2005, p.71)

"Hi everyone,
As Dana is about to embark on a 10-day detox programme (which I am also going to do) I thought it would be beneficial for you to be aware of what is happening and exactly why we are doing this.
Detoxification is simply getting rid of any harmful and foreign substances from the body. If our body is the temple of the Holy Spirit and we live in this modern age of chemicals, additives and preservatives, it makes sense that we should detox our body … This 10-day diet that we are going to begin on Easter Sunday is also going to be a faith journey for us as we seek God and ask Him for complete healing for Dana …
By following this diet we are putting faith into action …
Knowledge without action is a non-event. So we are going to go for it!!!
… Please pray believing prayers that we will see a miracle happen.
With love"

Mum sent that email out to our extended family. We knew full well that to be bathed in prayer during this step of faith was so important. We really were 'going for it'. I am so thankful for the huge blessing of a believing, loving, supportive family.

As an added encouragement, the verse for April on my wall calendar in my room read, *"My God will meet all your needs according to His glorious riches in Christ Jesus."* (Philippians 4:19, NIV)

Let's do it.

Day 1: Resurrection Sunday (4th April, 2010).

This is the day in which Christians across the earth celebrate that Jesus is alive. He rose from the dead after three days in the tomb, and for the next 40 days He went on to prove it to hundreds of people who were eye-witnesses of His resurrection before then ascending to heaven in clear view of His disciples. Jesus is still alive today. He is alive forever, and we have the promise of eternal life after death – if we *repent* of (turn away from) our sins and *believe* Jesus is the Son of God and has been raised from the dead. This truly is something to celebrate.

What a day to begin the Daniel's Diet detox!

Our first task...

'Upon rising' Psyllium husks and a glass of water ...

Wow. It looked like sawdust floating around in the glass. No matter how much you swirled it around the bits just kept on floating. Here goes ...

The 'sawdust' felt like tiny bits of wet cardboard dancing across my tongue as I attempted to swallow ...

Ughhh! That's gross! The flavour wasn't much better than wet cardboard either!

I think the only good thing about that experience is that there's one less of those to have now!

Eww.

Next ... about half an hour later it was time for 'Pre-breakfast'. Prunes in lemon juice. This should be ok. I like prunes. I don't mind the lemon flavour. Overnight we had soaked the prunes in a small amount of pure, unadulterated, simply squeeze the lemon on top of the prunes, lemon juice. Our instructions were to eat the prunes and then drink up the excess juice.

As I placed the first prune in my mouth my lips caught the edge of my fingers and the sourness of the lemon hit me with a force I was not expecting. Thankfully though as I started chewing the prune, the sweetness overcame the sourness ... mostly.

With each prune, the sour, acidic lemon taste grew stronger until finally it was time to drink the juice ... as I took a sip the glands in the back of my mouth became on full alert — they were shouting at me "Warning, warning, too sour! Warning, warning not coping!" Ohh the pain!

I have never experienced that before! The good news was that we were only doing 'prunes in lemon juice' every second day. One down. Four to go! Bring on breakfast!

Breakfast and morning tea were rather uneventful and lunch went over fairly well although we had a lot of leftover pumpkin! I suppose when you cook a whole baked pumpkin stuffed with vegetables it will be a lot of pumpkin! There is only so much pumpkin I could eat too. A few mouthfuls was (and is) truly my limit if I want to enjoy pumpkin. Anything beyond that starts to make me feel off. Yes, I was more than happy to donate the leftovers to the rest of the family.

By the time we had finished afternoon tea, Mum and I were surprisingly feeling very well satisfied. I wasn't sure I had much room left for dinner! This was a nice surprise as we had wondered if we would feel hungry whilst on the detox.

The dinner was "Warm chickpea salad". The problem was, the chickpeas were like little rocks! Dad and Rach were joining us for the dinner meals and Dad was adamant that these little rocks were that hard they could break a tooth! This experience scarred Dad for life – from this moment on he has always been cautious of chickpeas, believing no matter how you cook or prepare them, they will always be akin to trying to eat a marble.

Day 2: Monday 8th April.

Having made it through the psyllium husk 'upon rising' gut cleanser, Mum began to prepare our 'Pre-breakfast' "Refreshing cold vegetable drink". That is, a vegetable juice made of raw carrot, cauliflower, broccoli, celery, pumpkin and parsley blended up together. (Bridgeman, 2005, p.88)

I was hopeful. I like all those vegetables, and parsley is ok. Plus, think of all the amazing nutrients combined in the one refreshing drink.

Well, the name was half correct. Refreshing. No. Cold. Yes. Vegetable, definitely! Drink? That was the hard part. I really struggled to get it down ... And I thought the psyllium husks were bad! This was worse! So much so that we edited our meal plan table ... let's do more prunes in lemon juice and less refreshing cold vegetable drink!

Day 3: Tuesday 6th April.

After yesterday's vegetable blend disaster, I was a bit apprehensive about the 'Fruit porridge' breakfast for today. Pear or apple or strawberries, pumpkin seeds, Brazil nuts, banana or prunes, and LSA. (Bridgeman, 2005, p.91) I only recently started to eat nuts and seeds, so I was still getting used to the new flavours, but they were reasonably ok. How would they go in a 'porridge' with LSA and fruit? The name was not very enticing for me as I had tried porridge once or twice at my grandparents' house and did not enjoy it at all!

Into our mini food processor went all the ingredients and out came a sloppy, gritty mess.

Mum served it up and we prayed over it, then began the taste test. I placed the spoon tentatively in my mouth and relaxed a little as I realised it was actually not bad at all. A bit of a strange texture, but the flavour was fine. Phew.

Day 4: Wednesday 7th April.
The devotional verse for the detox Day 4 was: *"Therefore do not cast away your confidence, which has great reward. For you have need of endurance, so that after you have done the will of God, you may receive the promise."* (Hebrews 10:35-36). (Bridgeman, 2004, p.155)

Yes! Amen. May it be so, Father. In today's society we so often expect things instantly – we have microwaves to reheat food fast, we have express shipping when we order items, we have fast food takeaway places to get food quickly, we have planes that take us vast distances in a fraction of the time it would have taken to travel when only sail boats were around to cross oceans … and so on. Yet, here God reminds us that we need endurance. We need to do the will of God and then we may receive the promise … Obedient faith, then miraculous answers!

The first three days were behind us and we were going fairly well.

I had made it through the 'Upon rising' and 'Pre-breakfast' and after yesterday's success with breakfast I was looking forward to trying "Philip's breakfast". This was mixed berries, LSA, pumpkin seeds, lecithin and coconut milk (Bridgeman, 2005, p.18). That all sounded pretty safe. What was there not to like?

Well, I made an important, yet disappointing discovery. I do NOT like coconut 'milk'! I thought coconut milk would taste; I don't know … like coconut maybe? Nope!!! Nothing like it! (Looking back on this experience I'm wondering if Mum accidentally bought coconut water instead of coconut milk, as the coconut milk does have much more of a coconut flavour than what I remember trying to consume that day … and years later when I tried coconut water out of a fresh coconut it brought back memories of this breakfast! A strange, unenjoyable (for me) taste, nothing like the coconut flesh flavour!)

Whatever it was, it ruined the whole breakfast! Everything was drenched in the coconut 'milk' (or water?). Such a shame because the berries would have been great on their own. Cross that one off the list!

At least I knew the morning tea of corn thins with avocado, capsicum and (crunchy) chickpea dip would be nice. (Yes, corn thins were allowed as they were basically puffed corn with a little salt).

Day 5: Thursday 8th April.
By this day we were beginning to settle into the new routine of the seven 'meals' a day (Upon Rising, Pre-Breakfast, Breakfast, Morning Tea, Lunch, Afternoon Tea, Dinner) and we knew what to expect from some of the recipes as they were repeated. To end off the half-way point we enjoyed a fairly normal dinner of steamed vegetables with brown rice. Nothing exotic. Safe and delicious. Five days to go.

Day 6: Friday 9th April.
It was rather surprising that the 'Breakfast' of a banana wrapped in a cos lettuce leaf actually provided a tasty, satisfying meal.

Day 7: Saturday 10th April.

The devotional verse for today is: God… *"Who pardons all your iniquities; Who heals all your diseases."* (Psalm 103:2) (Bridgeman, 2004, p.156) This verse comes out of the Psalm which begins with *"Bless the LORD, O my soul; And all that is within me, bless His holy name! Bless the LORD, O my soul, And forget not all His benefits: Who forgives all your iniquities, Who heals all your diseases."* (Psalm 103:1-3). Every Christian knows the *"forgives all your iniquities"* part. But we wrestle or dismiss the very next phrase *"Who heals all your diseases"*. I suppose it may be an issue of faith (can He really heal anything?) or an issue of timing (when will the healing happen? Ultimately believers will be healed in eternity). I believe God CAN heal all diseases. I believe He WILL heal me of chronic fatigue… in this life.

Day 8: Sunday 11th April.

It has been a whole week. It is hard to believe that we are on Day 8 and we have actually done a week on this detox. I am so thankful Mum has taken this journey with me and I am believing this will be a huge step forward in getting healed fully.

Day 9: Monday 12th April.

The dinner tonight was Lentil Bolognaise and brown rice. It was so nice to have the bolognaise flavours. Something familiar, yet different. One day to go.

Day 10: Tuesday 13th April.

Having the final psyllium husk gut cleanser brought forth a sense of achievement and a real relief! By now the 'prunes in lemon juice' were handled well by my glands and the nuts and seeds mix for afternoon tea was quite enjoyable. Only a few weeks ago I never would have thought I would enjoy eating nuts and seeds!

Day 11: Wednesday 14th April.
We have completed the 10 days! Amazing!
The devotional verse for Day 11 was:
"Afterwards Jesus found him in the temple, and said to him, "See, you have been made well. Sin no more, lest a worse thing come upon you." (John 5:14) (Bridgeman, 2004, p.157)

The next few weeks saw us slowly reintroducing the good foods which were not part of the detox (the good meats, other grains, eggs, dairy and so on). Then once these good foods were reintroduced, I hoped to continue with this lifestyle of eating healthy, whole foods as much as possible. Philip calls it 'Daniel's Diet Lifestyle' (which is also the title of his book).
Let the Daniel's Diet Lifestyle journey begin.

Chapter 20: Walk by faith

After completing the Daniel's Diet detox, I gradually improved, gaining strength more and more. It certainly was not an instant healing during or right after the detox, but during the detox I felt the same or better than I had in the lead up to it and after it I never looked back. I continued to walk by faith and not by sight, though I was getting glimpses of what it would look like to be well again, and I desired to continue eating healthy anyway.

The Daniel's Diet Lifestyle is not meant to feel like you are on a temporary diet that you will finish someday and go back to eating whatever you like. Rather, if you can relearn that the word diet is just a name for what you eat, and you desire to eat healthy, whole foods, then it does become a lifestyle and not a strict plan to follow. It is a little like the Old and New Testament. God gave the Law as a tutor and a guardian to show people how to live until Jesus came with the New Covenant (see Galatians 3:23-25). Now for the Christian, the Law is written in our hearts and we desire to do what is right, so we fulfil the Law by living God's ways. What's right and wrong did not change, but we don't try to do it in our own strength now, we do it by the power of the Holy Spirit as a new creation in Christ with His love filling our heart. Similarly, what we should eat did not change, but now I have a desire to eat what is good, it is easy to say no to food that is not life-giving. I do not need a strict diet plan to follow. I have freedom to choose anything that is wholesome.

What does that look like practically? A lot less pre-packaged snacks. More home-baking with wholesome ingredients. Mostly not having dessert (unless it is a healthy version) as these are often full of non-life-giving ingredients. Staying away from processed deli meats and soft drinks. Choosing to eat the meats that God indicated were for eating in His Word and avoiding where possible the meats that are not designed for eating.

Is it possible? Yes. Thirteen and a half years later and going strong. I have learnt over the years that the Philip Bridgeman *Daniel's Diet Lifestyle* and *Daniel's Diet* books provided an excellent foundation but there was still much more to learn and I am still learning more about what is nourishing and what is detrimental for our bodies.

People who have not read the books or have not had a similar journey often find it hard to understand these things. It is hard for me to 'get in their shoes' and it is hard for them to 'get in my shoes'.

As I continued eating in this new way I would often be asked, "Are you allowed to have this?" My response would always be along the lines of, "Yes, but I am choosing not to." I would also use this Scripture to explain: in relation to a similar topic, it says *"All things are lawful [that is, morally legitimate, permissible], but not all things are beneficial or advantageous. All things are lawful, but not all things are constructive [to character] and edifying [to spiritual life]."* (1 Corinthians 10:23 AMP). So, it is perfectly reasonable to choose what is beneficial!

Sometimes there would be comments like "That must be so hard" or "You're so strong" or "You're so good". The truth is, in the vast majority of cases it is actually not hard at all.

Saying "No" is easy as I have no, or very little, desire for foods that I know are not good for me. It's that simple.

What was hard though, was disappointing family who had created special desserts and I would say "No thank you" and they would not understand why I would politely decline ... why I wouldn't get to enjoy their creation they had laboured over in love ... why I wouldn't have just a little bit because that's not going to hurt me.

So, after some time I decided to try 'a little' bit of some of these creations. I could see that it was really disappointing them and I figured it wouldn't hurt me too much to try a small bit for them. But the problem was, though everyone else loved the desserts, I would just get a headache or dizziness for about 20 – 30 minutes after a small taste. My body had adjusted to not having sugar spikes and to get one it was so obvious and not enjoyable at all. So, that experiment ended. It was not worth it. I did not desire the overly sweet foods and my body did not cope with them anymore anyway.

It also puzzled me that almost any kind of eating was catered for readily except for just genuinely wanting to eat healthy. Gluten free? No worries. Vegetarian? We will cater for you. Vegan? We'll make it work. Dairy free? We can do it. Allergic to (insert food here)? Leave it with us.

But ... No added sugar? It just wouldn't rate a mention. It was like it was unheard of.

No pork? What is wrong with you? – Don't you know we are living in the New Covenant?!

Hmm.

Yes, I know we are living in the New Covenant, but there is so much wisdom in the Old Testament for us to learn from. Pigs were listed as not for eating. They are scavengers (eat anything) and often carry many diseases – why shouldn't we choose to avoid them?

People who were kind of half paying attention to my journey would get all mixed up and excitedly say, "I've made you this gluten free, dairy free dessert" and I would politely say… "Wow, thank you. I can eat gluten and dairy though. Is there any sugar in it?" And often the answer would be a puzzled, "Yes" …

So, to those people who have done a bit of the food journey with me … I love you; I am sorry it has been hard to understand me … hopefully you are beginning to understand and appreciate it a bit more by now.

And for anyone wanting to go on this journey – despite those challenges I just mentioned, it really is worth it.

Five and a half months after the detox I reflected on where I was at. I wrote up a table of advantages and disadvantages to the Daniel's Diet Lifestyle I had been following since the detox. The advantages far outweighed the disadvantages. The only disadvantages were losing too much weight (not an issue for most people – I was just not all that big to start with), what to eat when eating out if I hadn't planned ahead, and misunderstanding from others.

The advantages were wonderful and numerous! More continuous energy levels, able to do a lot more during the day, feeling healthier, lost excess weight (which I had gained from not being able to do much exercise over the chronic fatigue affected years leading up to the detox), bowels regulated, nose unblocked, much less waking during the night, getting to sleep easier, no colds or flu during winter (unheard of for me!), did not get the sickness that so many people around me had, have begun to like a lot more foods, tastebuds enjoy a greater variety, more keen to try new things (as long as they are healthy), menstrual cycle periods are less painful and not as heavy, opportunity to share what I have learned to help others.

I also began to realise that in the Bible if people were healed, they would often be asked to test it out. When Jesus healed the man with a withered hand, He asked the man to stretch out his hand (see Matthew 12:9-13). When Jesus healed the 10 lepers, He asked them to go and show themselves to the priest (see Luke 17:11-19). When Jesus healed the paralysed man by the pool of Bethsaida, He asked him to pick up his mat and walk (see John 5:5-9). Can a paralysed man walk? Can a leper be healed on his way to a priest? Can a withered hand be stretched out? No. But Jesus asked them to by faith – and they were healed as they obeyed, there was proof of the healing as they stepped out in obedient faith. To me, that was an invitation to start trying things I would not have done because 'I don't have the energy'. So, I began to do more at church, I began to drive more and started to drive at night again if I needed to, I did more physical activity, and so on. And as I stepped out in faith, I was able to do these things.

Praise God!!

Chapter 21:
In the name of Jesus

So, are you healed now?"

It was 2012. I had been steadily improving since April 2010 when I did the Daniel's Diet detox and then continued with Daniel's Diet Lifestyle ever since. I was doing most things as if I was healed, but where was I truly at?

This question seemed to keep coming up with increasing frequency. How do I answer it honestly? What if I answer "Yes!" and then get another relapse? What if I answer "Yes" and then people expect everything of me which my body may not be ready for yet? What if I answer "No" but I actually am healed and then I am missing opportunities to give God the glory?

Honestly, I didn't know. Maybe I was? I was a lot better than before. But it had been nearly 5 years! It had been such a long time that I couldn't remember how I felt before chronic fatigue.

My answer was usually "I'm a lot better than I was". But I really did want to give people a definitive answer. I wanted to be able to say with confidence, "Yes, God has healed me! I do not have chronic fatigue anymore."

Then, Mum had an idea.

When I first got sick way back in June 2007, there were about five to seven warts that grew on the back of my right heel. They grew in a circle around a spot where I had had a wart frozen off many years prior but they were smaller than that one which had been frozen off. The doctor told us that warts are a sign that there is a virus active in the body.

When I had the relapse the summer of 2009/2010 more warts grew in the exact same spot. They filled in more of the circle around the same spot where the old wart had been before it was removed. About four more of them. Now I had somewhere between nine and eleven little warts in a circle on the back of my right heel.

"I'm going to pray that the warts disappear and when they do that will be a sign that you are healed!"

That sounded like a great idea to me. I was still a bit sceptical as to if God would answer that prayer, but I knew it was definitely worth a try and how cool would it be to see that take place ... and then I would have a definitive answer once God performed that sign, confirming that He had completed the miracle of healing me.

So, I joined Mum in praying for the warts to go as a sign that I was healed.

But wait a minute... are we allowed to ask God for a sign? Aren't we not meant to test God? Jesus rebuked the Pharisees for asking Him for a sign when He had already given them so many. Even so, He did give them one more sign He would perform... *"Then some of the scribes and Pharisees answered, saying, "Teacher, we want to see a sign from You." But He answered and said to them, "An evil and adulterous generation seeks after a sign, and no sign will be given to it except the sign of the prophet Jonah. For as Jonah was three days and three nights in the belly of the great fish, so will the Son of Man be three days and three nights in the heart of the earth."* (Matthew 12:38-40)

They tried it again later... *"Then the Pharisees and Sadducees came, and testing Him asked that He would show them a sign from heaven. He answered and said to them,*

"When it is evening you say, 'It will be fair weather, for the sky is red'; and in the morning, 'It will be foul weather today, for the sky is red and threatening.' Hypocrites! You know how to discern the face of the sky, but you cannot discern the signs of the times. A wicked and adulterous generation seeks after a sign, and no sign shall be given to it except the sign of the prophet Jonah." (Matthew 16:1-4).

They were blind to the signs Jesus had already shown them, but Jesus still gave them that one more sign to look for. There are also at least two stories in Scripture where God is happy with people asking Him for a sign to confirm something He has said: Gideon and King Hezekiah.

Here is Gideon's story:

"So Gideon said to God, "If You will save Israel by my hand as You have said— ³⁷ look, I shall put a fleece of wool on the threshing floor; if there is dew on the fleece only, and it is dry on all the ground, then I shall know that You will save Israel by my hand, as You have said." ³⁸ And it was so. When he rose early the next morning and squeezed the fleece together, he wrung the dew out of the fleece, a bowlful of water. ³⁹ Then Gideon said to God, "Do not be angry with me, but let me speak just once more: Let me test, I pray, just once more with the fleece; let it now be dry only on the fleece, but on all the ground let there be dew." ⁴⁰ And God did so that night. It was dry on the fleece only, but there was dew on all the ground." (Judges 6:36-40).

Whilst Gideon's sign was about confirming an assignment God had given him, amazingly King Hezekiah asked for a sign that he would be healed. Can you believe that? That is exactly what Mum and I were doing.

Here is King Hezekiah's story:

"And Hezekiah said to Isaiah, "What is the sign that the LORD will heal me, and that I shall go up to the house of the LORD the third day?"

⁹ Then Isaiah said, "This is the sign to you from the LORD, that the LORD will do the thing which He has spoken: shall the shadow go forward ten degrees or go backward ten degrees?"

¹⁰ And Hezekiah answered, "It is an easy thing for the shadow to go down ten degrees; no, but let the shadow go backward ten   degrees."

¹¹ So Isaiah the prophet cried out to the LORD, and He brought the shadow ten degrees backward, by which it had gone down on the sundial of Ahaz." (2 Kings 20:8-11)

Around the time I began to pray for the warts to go I started to see that when Jesus healed people, He didn't really pray for healing ... He would command people to do something they could not do before, or touch them and they would be healed; rather than ask the Father to do the healing. And if He was casting out a demon, He would command them to come out and they would. He said things like, *"Stretch out your hand"* (Matthew 12:13b), *"Pick up your mat and walk"* (John 5:8b), *"receive your sight"* (Luke 18:42b), *"be cleansed"* (to the leper) (Matthew 8:3b), *"be healed of your affliction"* (Mark 5:34b), *"Lazarus come forth"* (when raising Lazarus from the dead) (John 11:43b), *"Little girl, I say to you, arise"* (when raising the little girl from the dead) (Mark 5:41b), *"Come out of the man, unclean spirit!"* (see Mark 5:8b)

The apostles often followed Jesus' example in this, as rather than asking the Father for healing, they would lay hands on the sick, and they would command the person to do something in faith in the name of Jesus. There is power in His name and in having faith in Jesus. See Acts 3:1-8 and Acts 4:8-12. In Mark 16:18b, Jesus said that those who believe in Him *"will lay hands on the sick, and they will recover"*.

So, I began (quite awkwardly and tentatively) to command the warts to be gone, in Jesus' name as I placed my hand on them. I also continued to pray for God to remove the warts because we are encouraged to pray to God about everything (see Philippians 4:6-7), so I figured healing and signs of healing must fall into that category.

Tuesday July 17, 2012 I was drying off after my shower. 5 years, 1 month and 12 days after first getting sick. It was evening. As I went to rub the towel over my right foot, I suddenly realised that the warts were gone. ALL of them! Every. Single. One.

Gone!

What?!

Thank You Jesus! Thank You, Thank You, Thank YOU!!

I quickly got dressed, overwhelmed and excited and still processing it all.

"Mum!" I called out...

"Mum, come and have a look!"

Mum made her way upstairs and I grinned from ear to ear.

"Look, Mum" ...

I was sitting on the lounge. I bent my knee and turned my right foot towards Mum, pointing at my heel...

"They're gone!"

Mum gazed down at my right heel and the tears welled up in her eyes.

She looked at me with a heart full of gratitude and release. She began to thank God, and cry some more, and hug me, and be full of joy!

How good is God!

"Dad!" I called out.

"Look! The warts are all gone! All at once!"

Dad smiled and began to take it all in too.

"Rach! Come and see!"

We all rejoiced together.

Chapter 22:
Testify

Once those warts disappeared, I knew I had my answer. The healing has taken place. I am sure of this. I am confident.

I began to testify.

Now I was hoping people would ask me the question so I could share God's miracle with them!

There were so many opportunities to share! At church, at university, with extended family, with friends, then later on at work as well … it was great!

This was 11 years ago now and I can boldly proclaim that this healing has stood the test of time. I have had no further relapses and I have done things that would have been impossible if I still had any trace of chronic fatigue. I have worked full-time as a high-school teacher in a public school. I have gone on Youth Camps. I have travelled overseas on long-haul flights and explored other countries with a pace that some would describe as high intensity (holidays are for adventure, not for relaxing!). I am now a mother of a three-year-old and anyone who has gone through a pregnancy and raised a toddler knows how much energy that requires!! God is good. He is faithful.

What God has done for me; He can do for you, if that be His will. Your journey might look different, but He is all-powerful, all-loving and He knows what You need. I don't

www.ingramcontent.com/pod-product-compliance
Lightning Source LLC
Chambersburg PA
CBHW070804260726
48660CB00005B/1696